The Ultimate Mouth Manual

The Ultimate Mouth Manual

The Keys to Dental Health

SECOND EDITION

Lee N. Sheldon, DMD
Matthew E. Sheldon, DMD

with Rebecca Hunton, MD and Colin Richman, DMD

Pritz Publishing
Melbourne, FL 32935

978-0-578-14008-7

Printed in the United States of America

DISCLAIMER
The material in this book is intended to provide overall information only. The author and publisher assume no responsibility for the correct or incorrect use of this material, and no attempt should be made to use any of this information without the approval and guidance of your doctor. Fictitious names have been given to some of the patients mentioned to preserve patient confidentiality.

Contents

This book is dedicated to Sylvia "Sonnee" Sheldon.
There was no better Mom or Grandma.

Foreword to the Second Edition

IN my position as the director of an Advanced Education in General Dentistry (AEGD) residency program, it is our goal to provide experience and instruction in current materials, techniques and procedures to our residents, and most become very successful quickly upon graduation. I am very familiar with the joy in seeing a son or daughter follow in our footsteps and attend dental school, as one of my boys went to dental school, even was one of my residents for a year, and we're still very close colleagues and friends! The first edition of *The Ultimate Mouth Manual* by Dr. Lee Sheldon was given to me by his son, Matt, who was also one of my residents. On the cover, Matt was credited as "with Matthew Sheldon, DMD". This second edition represents the excellence seen in the younger Sheldon during and after his AEGD, and it is obvious that he and the elder have partnered to become an awesome team to be admired. I believe this to be exciting, and this is only a hint at what is to come from them in the future! On the cover of the second edition, both Dr. Lee and Matt Sheldon have equal billing.

The first edition was a refreshing, informative common sense approach to explaining many areas around periodontics and related systemic conditions that provide valuable education for clinicians, students and patients alike. Therein lay a clear manner in which to educate patients to raise success rates of home care and compliance. And when Matt joined with his father and they began sharing clinical treatment of patients together, something exemplary began to happen. Not only are they extremely compatible, they are professionally highly motivated, knowledgeable and enthusiastic about contributing to the dental community. They are an ideal team of a periodontist and general dentist, able to provide nearly all areas of dentistry to their patients in the same office.

I thought the first edition was uniquely amazing. Why hadn't someone explained these things like this when I was in dental school? And the topics and information was very current and all inclusive. Fast forward less than two short years – Matt joins his dad after his residency, they share their drive to learn and improve their patient care, and the second edition is born. This new book contains all the information from the first, with some update modifications, but adds many topics related to current concepts in comprehensive care for the general dentist. Again, it is written in language understood by lay people, yet contains valuable, accurate information for clinicians as well. Current topics such as bleaching, xerostomia, foreign dental care, implant options, cosmetic treatment and the connection with systemic disease and the oral cavity are presented extremely well. I read the new edition with great interest, and am thoroughly impressed. I intend to make sure my own son gets a copy. Dr. Lee Sheldon should be very proud – what the Sheldon's have is rare and envied. I believe that all general dentists should have this book and that it be available in all waiting rooms. If all dental schools taught like this and all dentists practiced like this, it would be a perfect world! Enjoy the book, and share it with colleagues and patients!

Charles W. Wakefield, DDS, MAGD, ABGD
Dallas, Texas

Foreword

IT is a great honor for me to write this foreword for Dr. Lee Sheldon's book, *The Ultimate Mouth Manual.* My wife Maureen and I had the pleasure of meeting Lee and his wife Eleanor at the University of Connecticut, School of Dental Medicine, where we were both enrolled as periodontal residents. From our early encounters, it became evident that Lee was a talented and inquisitive dentist, perpetually questioning the status quo and always looking for a better way to treat his patients more effectively and with greater predictability. This was because Lee entered our residency program with marked personal and professional maturity for someone who had only recently graduated dental school. We completed our residency programs and Lee and Eleanor moved to Florida to establish a home and a practice. However, we have continued to collaborate throughout the years, always questioning dogma, looking for a 'better way' of delivering reliable care, and challenging each other to move to an advanced level of cost effective treatment for our patients.

Lee might truly be described as a both an innovator and a maverick in the field of Periodontics, perpetually seeking truth over accepted belief through contemporary scientific research. When found, he then effectively implements those new treatment concepts which will best benefit his patients, into his armamentarium of available therapies.

This book is a synthesis of Lee's lifetime work effort. It reflects his growth, both as a human being as well as a clinical periodontist. The book is a valuable resource for existing and potential patients, dental professionals, periodontal residents and dental students. Although the content is technically accurate and timely, it has been written so personally that it provides its readers with an accurate assessment of the diverse therapeutic activities a clinical periodontist is involved in on a daily basis. It reflects Lee's very personal approach to understanding the science of both Periodontics and Implant Dentistry, as well as how he utilizes both the art and the science of this knowledge to provide his patients with contemporary and, most importantly, predictable dental care.

Despite Lee's immersion in his professions, he and his wife have never waivered on their commitment to their family or their community. Together they have raised and educated three wonderful children while also devoting themselves to community leadership and responsible civic citizenship. This book demonstrates that selflessness on many levels.

It is with great pleasure that I recommend this book, both as an educational resource, and as an example of a person who is truly committed to his profession and to his patients.

ENJOY!!

Colin S. Richman DMD

Atlanta, Georgia.

OUR PHILOSOPHY

Why I work with Dr. Lee Sheldon

IT'S often that I have to reveal the human side of Dr. Sheldon when I am explaining to patients their recommended treatment and its cost. This is actually a really hard thing to do for some in my field. On a daily basis, there is always a patient who makes a comment like, "What kind of car am I buying Dr. Sheldon this year?" or "Which of Dr. Sheldon's kids am I putting through college this time?" and to an assistant in a different office, it may be the part of her job to "act" or "lie" or "pretend." I am SO glad I don't have to work at those offices.

I have been working with Dr. Sheldon for a very long time, and one thing that makes me feel so good on my drive home is that I can honestly say I feel good about what I do, and who I do it for. Without a doubt, I know when I sign someone up for treatment, I am getting ready to make someone very, very happy and improve his or her quality of life. It is so easy to sit with patients and present plans when I know what I am suggesting are honest, long-term, "this is going to work or your money back" plans. I have seen Dr. Sheldon turn patients away and send them to a dentist that would better suit their needs. I have seen Dr. Sheldon insist that patients take care of medical issues before they come back in for dental needs. I have seen him spend hours with patients to give them health and personal guidance to get them through difficult times in their lives. I have seen him come in early, work through lunch, stay after hours and on weekends, and even cancel an entire day of scheduled patients to help someone in need.

So when I am working with patients on a daily basis, and the question comes up of "Why this office? Why so much money? Why Dr. Sheldon?" I can proudly say, "Dr. Sheldon cares about you and the success of your treatment. He has the skills and the technology to make sure the treatment he has recommended works and will be successful. He takes care of his patients and stands behind his work. He is worth every penny you will invest, and you will be so happy you did it when you are all done." I KNOW what Dr. Sheldon has done for me and I KNOW what he will do for his patients. I have no problems sharing with my patients the absolute pleasure I have working for Dr. Sheldon. I do love coming to work and I do love doing what I do.

Danyel Joyner
Office Manager

What I think of Dr. Sheldon

1. Dr. Sheldon is the greatest periodontist in the world.
2. His tissue grafts are a work of art.
3. He thinks about your overall heath not just your mouth.
4. He is always very honest to you even if you don't want to hear it.
5. He cares a lot about his staff, at work or at home.
6. He remains on the cutting edge of the profession through constant education.
7. He uses the most advanced technology.
8. His ethics are beyond reproach.
9. His chair-side manner is awesome.
10. He gives continually to the community in time and donations.

Rebecca Caudill
Lead Dental Hygienist for over 27 years

How I Feel about Being a Dentist

DENTISTRY isn't a commodity, and I believe that I, as your dentist, can make a difference in more than just your mouth.

Your overall health is my interest, whether you are dentally healthy and need wellness advice or are a dental cripple and need rehabilitation. It is my job to improve your oral health and, as a result, your general health.

My responsibility is to you, not your insurance company, not even your other dentist as a first priority, but to you. Nor do I feel responsibilities to other industries whose tenets may conflict with your overall health and who, at worst, may profit from your failure.

My job is to give you direction as well as a total dental health plan that, if followed, will give you successful results in regards to your mouth and, as such, your total health.

I need your communication, your participation, and your contribution. But most of all, I need your commitment. This is our journey, and as long as we both agree, I will guide you, always making your needs my first priority.

Lee Sheldon

Develop a Relationship with your Health Care Provider

Dr. Lee Sheldon

THIS morning, Sunday, I received a call from Rosemary, a long time patient of mine. She was sorry to bother me on a Sunday, but she had broken a tooth and wanted to make arrangements to see me on Monday. I asked her if it was hurting her. It wasn't, and it was in the back of the mouth where no one could see it.

What was neat is that Rosemary was comfortable calling me on a Sunday. Lest you think that this is a bother to me, it is not. My patients respect my time and don't abuse the privilege of having my cell phone number. Within a couple of hours, my wife was able to check on when I had a slot open. She called Rosemary and I will see her tomorrow. If Rosemary had an infection or was in pain, I would have seen her on a Sunday.

Why am I even telling you this story? It is because dentists in private practice want to and are happy to hear from patients with whom they've developed a relationship. We don't treat patients as a commodity. We treat patients as friends. They've chosen us. We nurture that relationship and as that relationship develops, more and more trust develops as well.

In the current day of being on the "right plan," of finding plans with perceived "discounts," a significant segment of the population ignores the corporate sales pitches and instead chooses a relationship with their health care practitioner. And there are many health care practitioners, not only dentists, who want to develop relationships with patients. It isn't about money. We expect to be paid. It's more than that. It's the hugs, it's the appreciation, it's the knowledge that we are making a difference in a person's life.

The private practitioner, if he or she is good at it, thinks about what can be done to make that practice better, to be more valuable to the patient. The private practitioner has the flexibility to make decisions on that basis. There's no insurance company, no government entity, that will interfere with the private practitioner. And when there are no third parties standing in the way, the doctor/patient relationship thrives.

Many of my colleagues in medicine are envious of the position that we have in dentistry, of the fact that we can call our own shots. We don't have to justify our recommendations to a third-party payer. We make the decision with the patient. The patient can ask for alternatives, of how we can extend treatment out to make it more affordable, and together we work out a plan that will help the patient thrive in whatever way the patient chooses.

So in these days of battling about what the best healthcare plan is, let's bring it back to basics. Let's decide who we want to be with, who we can trust, and develop more relationships as Rosemary and I have. Health care will be better for it.

The Good Old Days of Dentistry

FOR those of us who are old enough to remember Leave It to Beaver when it was in its first run, let's review where dentistry was and where it is now. Here's what I remember: my dentist gave me a choice if I wanted to be numb or not. It was five dollars extra for that shot. My mom paid it. The drill was connected to a pulley. I'd watch the frayed part of that twine travel up and down while my head rattled to the beat of the drill. The water in the sink made those concentric revolutions. I'd try to spit right down the hole in the middle. Everyone wore white. I climbed up in the chair. The assistant adjusted those two little disks on the back of my head. She took a couple of x-rays and then went out for what seemed like an eternity getting those things developed. Then the dentist walked in and readjusted the same headrest that the assistant had just set. When I got all done, I climbed out of the chair and went behind the secretary's desk where there was a small box where I could pick out a toy. Now those were the days.

Fast forward to today. We have virtual teeth being placed on virtual models that are created by computer and CT Scans. We're taking fewer impressions as the age of goop is declining and being replaced with scanned images of our mouths instead. The images are e-mailed to a lab that creates accurate models of our mouths from those scans, or the images allow the dentist to design and mill a crown right in the office.

I placed my first implant on May 16, 1986. Implants used to come in one length and three widths. I used to have to cut them to the correct length, smooth them, and resterilize them all in a single surgical procedure. Imagine how long that procedure took. Now I do virtual surgery on the computer; e-mail the image of the virtual surgery to the lab, which makes me a guide that I can temporarily attach to the teeth; preselect the implant; and often place the implant without making an incision. We can then scan the implant and create an abutment (portion that fastens the crown to the implant) customized to the patient's gum tissue and surrounding tooth position and at the same time make the final crown for the implant—truly amazing and so much easier for both patient and dentist.

Long ago, some patients would hear that there is "not enough bone" for an implant. That problem is hardly ever seen any more. The dental CT scan can uncover bone that would never be seen in conventional x-rays. If there is still not enough bone, we have bone powders, putties, blocks, growth factors harvested from your platelets, and stem cell attractants all successfully replacing missing bone. Missing soft tissue? We have freeze-dried skin, membranes made of pericardium, growth factors, and the latest: cells grown in tissue culture that stimulate the body to replace missing gum tissue.

Technology is giving us more opportunities to live our dental lives comfortably. I wonder what the next fifty years will bring.

DIAGNOSIS

What to Look for in a Dental Examination

THERE is no shortage of new, innovative dental techniques to enhance your dental experience, your ability to chew, and your smile. But today, let's get back to basics and talk about what you should look for in a dental examination.

We grew up understanding that if there is a cavity, it needs to be fixed. This is "single-tooth" dentistry. However, as we've grown older, we may have lost teeth, had teeth crowned, broken teeth, had gum disease, gum recession, etc. Changes in the relationships between teeth occur as a result. It's for those reasons that our dental examinations should be more detailed. A full oral care plan should be developed, even if it may be months or years before it can be completed. A good plan can save money and help preserve your dental health.

For most who visit my practice, their dental deterioration is advanced. That doesn't mean that I'm not happy to see the "early" cases. I am. If I can help prevent a patient from becoming an advanced case, I love to do that. However, if you have had dental work done and redone, if you have given up on dentistry in general, or if you have worn dentures for years and find them to be more than a nuisance, then you are the typical patient in my office.

There is a depth to the examination that, in my opinion, is necessary for the advanced dental case. Some of these recommendations apply to the routine dental case as well, depending upon the need.

The following is a checklist of my examination recommendations when you are seeking dental care:

- A full periodontal examination, including periodontal probing, to determine the amount of bone support for a tooth, the degree of gum recession to determine the amount of root surface that's exposed, the thickness of the gum tissue, and tooth mobility.

- A full dental examination which looks at tooth decay, worn fillings and crowns that may be leaking, cracks and microfractures, and loss of enamel at the gum line.
- Full mouth dental x-rays. I want to be a bit careful here. The amount of radiation required for these x-rays is extremely small. However, it is still radiation. The greater your disposition to dental disease, the more important x-rays become.

The three examinations above should give you and your dentist an understanding as to the long-term risk for each tooth. After all, you don't want to spend a lot of money on a tooth that has a high risk of being lost.

- Bite relationship. Not only should you know how your teeth line up, you should also know which teeth touch and which don't. For the most part, all teeth should touch when you close your mouth.
- Joint and muscle assessment. Does your jaw pop or grind when you open or close your mouth. If so, why, and what can be done to reduce the chances of further joint damage?
- CT scan. A CT scan gives your dentist a three-dimensional view of your jaw. On a positive note, a CT scan often finds "hidden" bone that may not be seen on a traditional x-ray. And as a traditional x-ray shows the bone in only two dimensions, a CT scan can show bone volume, an essential piece of data when doing dental implants. The Cone Beam Dental CT Scan exposes the patient to only about 2% of the radiation of a traditional CT scan.
- Study models. For complex cases, impressions of your teeth and models of your mouth are made so that your dentist can look at your mouth from every different direction.

The more complex your case, the more essential these diagnostic elements become; but make no mistake about the fact that diagnosis should precede treatment. *The most expensive part of dentistry is redoing a dental procedure.* A little bit of planning can go a long way toward decreasing your costs and improving your results through effective, comprehensive dental treatment.

Diagnosis: One of the Keys to Success in Treatment

IMAGINE repairing a roof without knowing where the leak was. Or imagine changing a recipe without knowing the original recipe. How about creating a football defense without planning on the offense? Or treating an illness without doing some diagnostic tests first? And that's where we have made a lot of progress in dentistry—understanding that periodontal disease, tooth decay, and other oral diseases are actually diseases.

Diseases have causes, and the diseases of the mouth are mostly bacterially related. Specific bacteria have been identified that cause the most severe destruction of bone support. There is a good way to test to see if you have those bacteria. A simple saliva sample can be sent to the laboratory to identify how pathogenic your bacteria are.

The bacteria are one side of the equation. The second side is your ability to fight disease. The source of that ability is called the immune system. The immune system is created from a system of white blood cells that circulate in our bodies. When we're younger, we usually have great immune systems. We can roll around in the dirt, eat some of the unhealthiest foods, and we are usually not attacked by disease. If we are, we heal very quickly. That's the character of a healthy immune system.

We always have bacteria. Even having the worst bacteria, a healthy immune system can fight it. However, if the number of bad bacteria goes beyond a certain threshold, we can no longer fight it. Therefore, we not only need to identify the type of bacteria, but we also need to determine how much of that type of bacteria we have in our mouths.

There's a third aspect of disease, and that is our genetic susceptibility to it. If we have a particular combination of genes, we may be more likely to get a disease.

Wouldn't it be good to know about the bacteria that we have so that we can treat the disease most effectively? Wouldn't it be nice to know our genetic susceptibility? Such tests are available today. With a simple saliva sample, we can learn about the bacteria in your mouth. We can determine the quantity of such bacteria and we can learn about our genetic ability to fight it. With such information at hand, your treatment course can be scientifically charted, which will improve the effectiveness of treatment and give you a better chance to save your teeth. Such information also allows us to better determine your ability to heal after surgery and therefore better tailor your treatment.

X-Rays

WANT to know a secret? You think more of x-rays than we do. Not a week goes by when I don't hear the questions "What does the x-ray show?" or the more accusing "Didn't that show up in the x-ray?" We need x-rays, but they often don't show as much as we'd like.

X-rays provide a way to see pathology that we can't feel with our instruments or see with our enhanced vision. X-ray diagnosis is dependent upon three variables: (1) the quality of the x-ray, (2) the ability of the x-radiation to actually detect the problem, and (3) the ability of the doctor to see the problem on the x-ray.

The quality of today's dental x-rays is actually quite good. With the advent of digital radiography, we have the ability to magnify the x-ray image. It's amazing what happens when the small, traditional x-ray film, which is only an inch-and-a-half long, is instead replaced by an image that is projected on a thirty-seven–inch video screen. Not only can I see the image better, so can the patient.

The ability of the x-ray to detect the problem is a bit more difficult to explain. The x-ray beam needs to penetrate the tooth structure in order to show an image. The harder the substance, the whiter it shows up on an x-ray. So enamel is on the lighter side. Dentin is grayer. Tooth decay, which is soft, shows up as a darker image. But if there is a metallic crown on the tooth, the metal reflects the x-ray. X-rays don't penetrate metal, so anything that's under a metal crown can't be seen on the image. Pathology, which shows up as a darker structure, can be blocked by a lighter structure such as a root surface, so we can't see that pathology. A CT scan shows multiple images in different planes and is often better for identification of pathology. The three-dimensional CT scan allows us to see volume and particularly thickness of bone, which is critical to assessing the volume necessary for a dental implant.

Our ability to read the x-ray comes with training and experience. Despite the fact that I've been doing this for a long time, I often send images to an oral and maxillofacial radiologist for his interpretation, particularly for pathology cases.

As good as x-rays might be, they don't always tell the whole story. Years ago, I saw a gentleman who was missing all of his teeth, had a severely resorbed jaw, and couldn't chew. I referred him for a CT scan and found room for only two dental implants. Two dental implants are far better than none, but four dental implants would improve his chewing ability immensely. I then operated on the patient and found enough room for the four dental implants that he had hoped for.

X-rays are great, but they are not the entire diagnosis. Together with some of the advanced imaging technology available today as well as experience and sound clinical judgment, they can be an excellent tool in helping your dentist make a better diagnosis.

PERIODONTAL SOLUTIONS

Why You Get Gum Disease

HAVE you been put on the guilt trip? That's right. The plaque guilt trip abounds. Your gums bleed a little, and the hygienist looks at you and says, "You're not flossing well enough." And worse, "If you don't do any better, Dr. X will have to send you to the periodontist." Ah, a fate worse than death—being sent to the periodontist. Is it any wonder that people walk into my office frightened? I'll bet you're a little frightened, too. That's okay. We're often frightened of the unknown. Here's what our patients have said, just for a little reassurance.

Katherine states, "*When I first went to Dr. Sheldon, I had severe periodontal disease; so much so that I needed a bone replacement. Dr. Sheldon did an excellent job in replacing that bone. I continue to see Dr. Sheldon, and today after two years, I am doing just great. I continue to have my teeth cleaned and checked often and I have not needed to have any more bone replacements.*"

Maria says, "*I keep returning to Dr. Sheldon's office for cleaning because of the thoroughness of his staff. I had terrible gum problems until I started coming to Dr. Sheldon. My gums are healthy now, thanks to Dr. Sheldon and Rebecca.*"

Carl says, "*I've been coming to Dr. Sheldon since 1983 and he has done everything possible that could be done to rebuild and get my mouth in shape. I am glad he is younger than I am because I don't want him to retire. I have had repeated procedures done and Dr. Sheldon always follows up that evening by calling me. I find him and his staff very friendly, knowledgeable, professional, and they make you feel very comfortable. I highly recommend Dr. Sheldon and his staff to anyone.*"

Plaque is the initial cause of periodontal disease. However let's be clear about the disease. From watching the commercials, you'd think that everyone is running around with periodontal disease. Well, they aren't. About 30% of the people in this country have periodontal disease (periodontitis) that causes loss of the bone support for a tooth. The rest of us have gingivitis, a mild swelling of the gums, but no bone loss.

The commercials talk about toothbrushes that control gingivitis, toothpastes that control gingivitis, mouthwashes that control gingivitis, water pics that control gingivitis—you name it. They have all kinds of things that control gingivitis. Over 90% of us have gingivitis. You figure it out. Ninety percent have gingivitis; 30% have periodontitis. They never advertise anything that controls periodontitis. In other words, they can treat something that doesn't really cause a major problem, but the major problem is really not controlled by these products. Sound a little fishy? Well, if you can sell it, market it, which is exactly what all these manufacturers have done; they've invented products. They might be good products, but they won't get to the source of your periodontal disease. Oh yes, there is one thing. It's a pill. There's always a pill. This pill helps to prevent your connective tissues from going through the normal processes of breakdown and repair. It's advertised for periodontal disease, but it is not specific to periodontal problems. It works for only very specific forms of periodontal disease. I have been using the same medications for years with good results in only a small subset of patients with periodontal disease. It has already been cautioned against for people who have lung problems. The reason for this is that the pill interferes with normal tissue repair. Who knows what other precautions will be discovered? This pill should be reserved for the most severe cases that don't respond to good, routine periodontal treatment.

What are the leading causes of periodontitis (loss of bone support)?

1. Genetics
2. Smoking
3. (and a distant 3 at that) Plaque

Having a family history of periodontitis makes you more prone to getting periodontitis. If you're a smoker, you've already been beaten up about smoking with regard to other health problems. Now you have one more health problem that's related to smoking. Sorry, I only report the data.

If you're prone to periodontal disease due to genetics and smoking, what can a periodontist do? Well, he or she can't change your genetics. I hope that you'll stop smoking. While genetics and smoking make you more prone to the disease, the disease itself is fueled by bacteria below the gum line called plaque, and it's plaque that's the only thing we can control in the office setting. Plaque becomes hardened on the root of the tooth below the gum line. That hardened plaque is called calculus. Calculus is rough and collects more plaque. The plaque and calculus need a place to hide out, so they dissolve a little of the bone below the gum line, hide and do their thing, and dissolve a little more of the bone. That area where the bone used to be but is now a mass of jelly-like tissue against the root surface is called a pocket. As the pocket becomes deeper and deeper, the tooth can loosen. The bigger the pocket, the looser the tooth will become.

Once that plaque-fueled infection starts, we have to remove that plaque and calculus. That's the only way the pocket will heal. For a discussion on how we do that, please go to the chapters on non-surgical and surgical treatment.

The Different Types of Gum Disease

LET'S go over the different types of periodontal disease. By the way, periodontal comes from two words, *perio*–around and *dont*–tooth. If we're looking at periodontal problems, we're looking at areas around the tooth or on the outside of the tooth. What's on the outside of the tooth? Well, if you look under the gum line, there's the root of your tooth, there's the bone around the root, and fibers called ligaments to connect the root to the bone. By the way, the root is not the same as *root canal. The root canal is a tube that goes through the center of the root and has nerves and blood vessels within it called the "pulp." When the pulp dies or becomes highly inflamed, a procedure called a "root canal" is done to take the bad pulp out of the tooth (please see the chapters, "Is it Always Correct to Save a Tooth" and "Before You Do that Root Canal"). Take a look at the picture on the next page.*

The common types of periodontal disease are the following:

Chronic Periodontitis—the usually gradual loss of the ligament and bone support for the tooth. It creates a pocket that is occupied by bacterial plaque and calculus.

Acute periodontitis—a painful swelling of the gum tissue caused by bacteria that's trapped below the gum line.

Gingivitis—the non-painful swelling of the gum tissue without any underlying bone or ligament damage.

Apical periodontitis—the inflammation and loss of bone support at the end of the root caused by a dead nerve within the root canal of the tooth.

The word, periodontal, means "around the tooth." Therefore, periodontal disease refers to the gums, ligaments, and bone which are around the tooth.

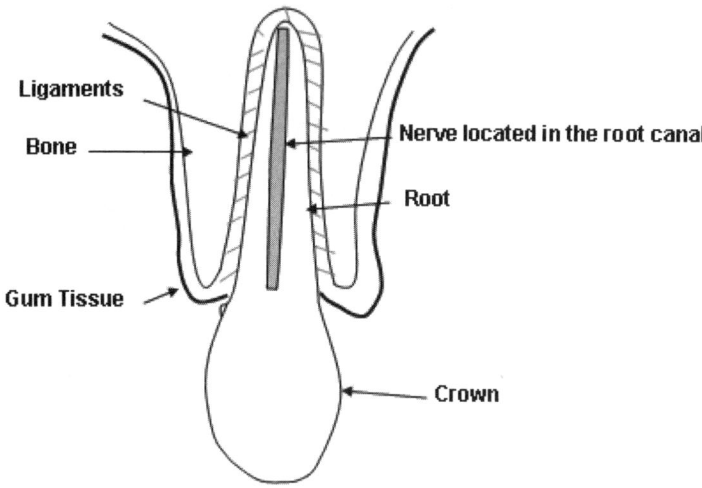

Let's look at the progression of chronic periodontitis.

Plaque bacteria accumulate on the tooth around the gum line.

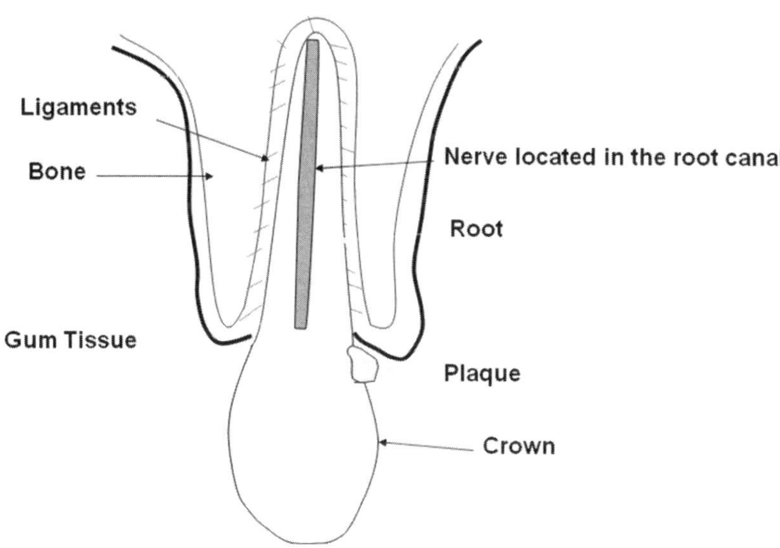

The gum tissue swells and bleeds a bit. This is called gingivitis.

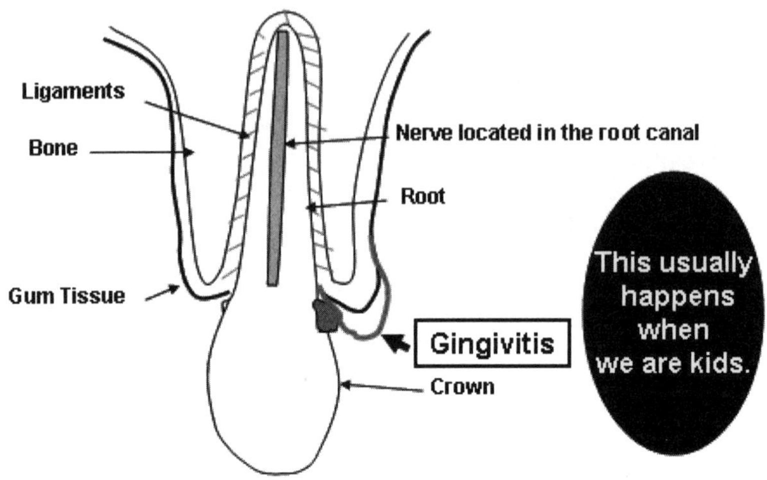

The bone starts to change and disappear.

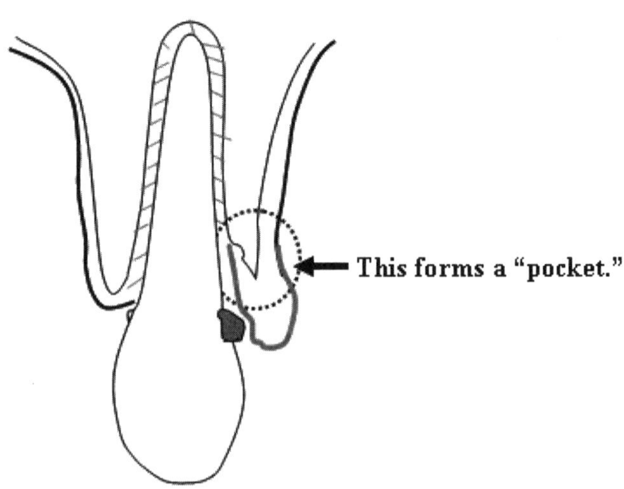

It is not unusual for bleeding to stop because all of the inflammation is now inside the pocket which usually isn't reached with the toothbrush or floss.

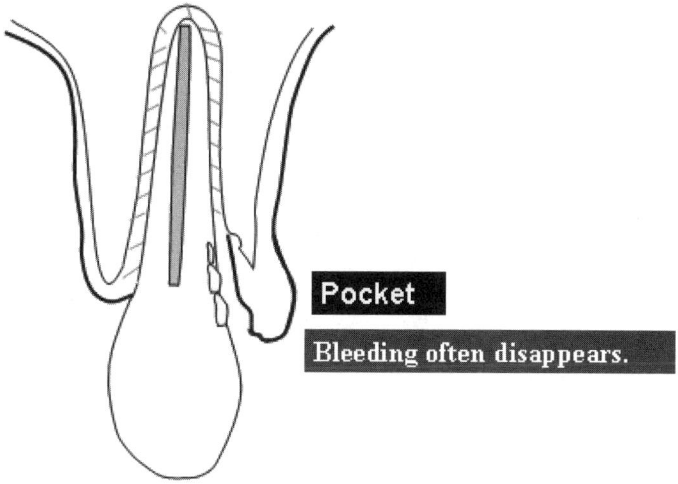

The depth of the pocket is measured with a small ruler called a probe.

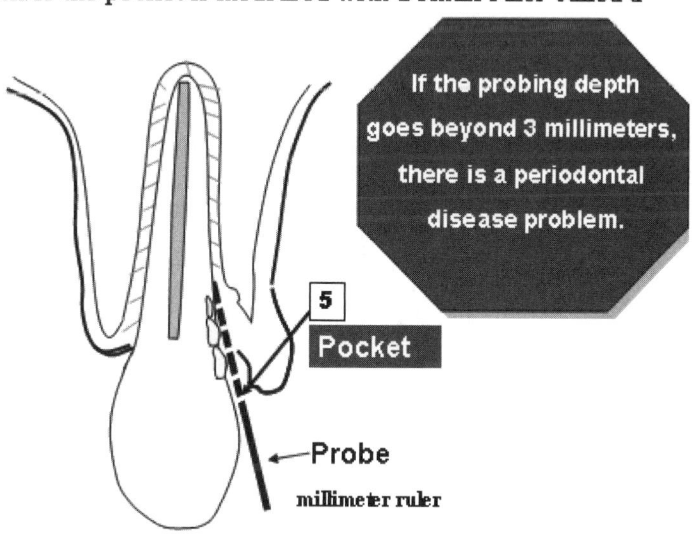

The plaque fills with minerals and blood. This is called calculus.

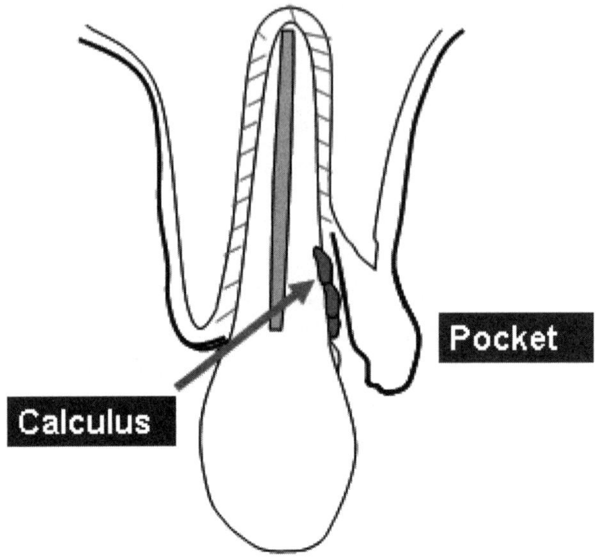

The pocket gets deeper.

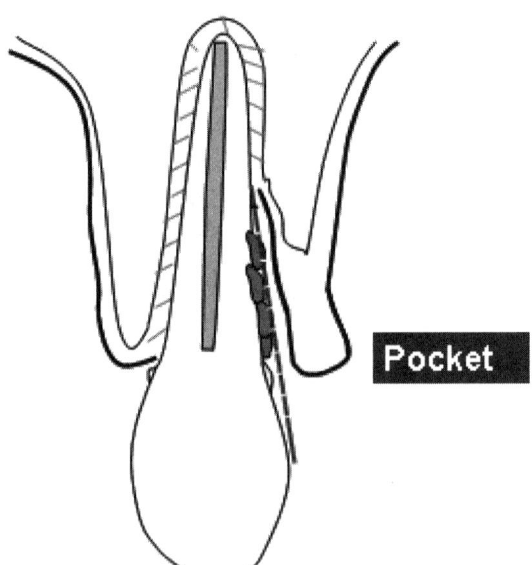

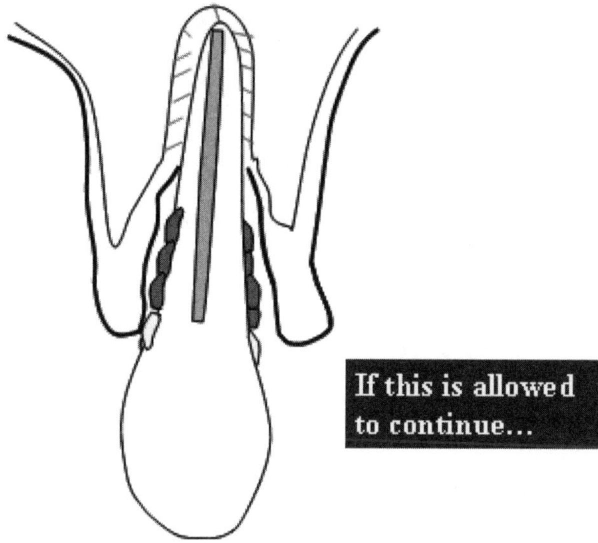
If this is allowed
to continue...

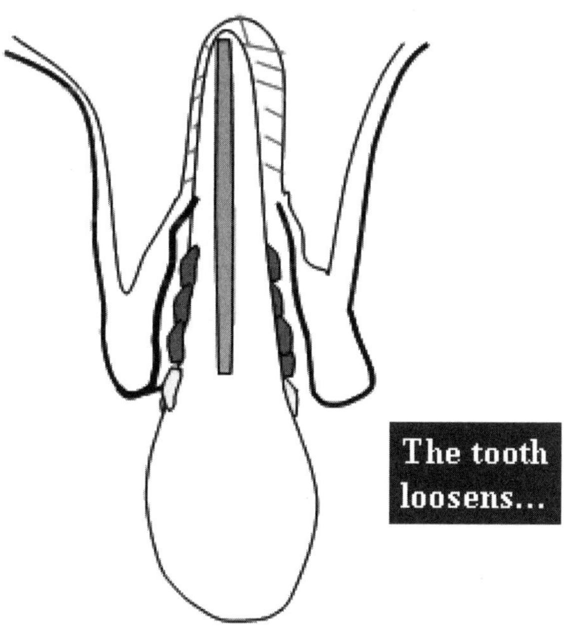
The tooth
loosens...

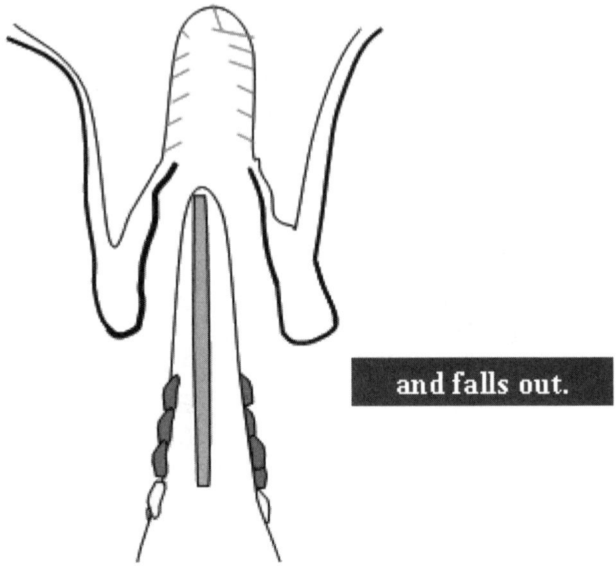

Case Story

Mark was 30 years old. He had come to the office all the way from Tampa. He had been told by two doctors that he would have to have all of his teeth taken out. I examined him and saw that he had very severe periodontal disease and a lot of bone loss. While extractions may have been a good option, the teeth were still firm, so there was a chance that they could be saved. When Mark came in, he was frightened that he would lose his teeth. What was interesting was that although he had an aggressive periodontal disease, it was well-controlled with antibiotics, and it is amazing how much bone came back with just non-surgical periodontal therapy and appropriate antibiotic therapy. He ended up losing only one tooth. We followed him for about four years and then he resumed his treatment in Tampa. This is just testimony to the fact that if the disease is identified and proper therapy is given in an aggressive situation, the bone can come back. This doesn't happen with everybody, and it's most likely to happen if the teeth are still firm and one is still young.

Periodontal Disease—Truth and Misconceptions

LET'S talk about periodontal disease, the truth and the misconceptions.

Here's the misconception: you or your dentist missed something so as a result you now have a disease. Could that be true? Only if you believe that people get heart attacks because their doctors miss something or people get cancer because their doctors miss something, or people get Alzheimer's because their doctors miss something, and so on.

The fact is that periodontal disease falls into a class of diseases known as chronic degenerative disease. Chronic means that it's continuing. Degenerative means that it's breaking down something, and that's what's happening. The critical attachment fibers between your teeth and your bone are breaking down.

Here are some of the factors that cause periodontal disease.

- Bacterial plaque—that's the soft bacteria that grows on the teeth. It's there whether we eat or not, and it needs to be removed at least once every twenty-four hours. That's your job, and the better that you do your job, the better the control of this factor of the disease
- Calculus—that's hardened plaque that migrates below the gum line. It's rough and accumulates more plaque, causing more loss of bone support. Why? The bone doesn't want to be anywhere near the plaque and calculus. Calculus can be removed only by a dentist or dental hygienist.
- Bad diet—There are so many bad foods that we eat. They are associated with all of the chronic degenerative diseases. The best part of our diets is a large variety of fresh fruits and

fresh vegetables. The larger the variety the better. The World Health Organization states flatly that 85 percent of cancers can be avoided and half are caused by nutritional deficiencies. Five to nine or more servings of fruits and vegetables are the standard way to protect yourself from any chronic degenerative disease, including periodontal disease.

- Genetics—People are genetically predisposed to certain diseases, but genetic *predisposition* does not mean genetic *expression.* If you do good things for yourself, you likely won't get the disease.
- Smoking—Yes, we do see that more smokers have periodontal disease than non-smokers by a wide margin. A recent study shows that the most periodontally damaging bacteria flourish in the mouth of a smoker.

So you see, it isn't just one factor at all that causes periodontal disease and therefore the best treatment for the disease addresses all of the above factors.

There are also times when a laboratory study of your bacteria is necessary because periodontal disease can be caused by one or a combination of eleven different types of bacteria. Identification of the bacteria gives you a chance to have the right antibiotic to kill that bacteria. We don't usually need or use antibiotics, but if the disease remains uncontrolled after treatment, then that laboratory study is invaluable.

With the right combination of diagnosis, coaching, professional instrumentation, and diet, you too can save your teeth. The earlier you do it, the better the opportunity.

Nutrition and Periodontal Disease

THE area that doctors and researchers are currently studying very carefully is chronic inflammation. In fact, chronic inflammation may very well be the common link to all of the chronic degenerative diseases—arthritis, heart disease, some forms of cancer, asthma, Alzheimer's disease, diabetes, and periodontal disease, to name just a few.

Periodontal disease is that disease which causes the loss of the supporting bone for the teeth. Also known as pyorrhea and gum disease, periodontal disease robs the person of his or her teeth, resulting in loss of mouth function, loss of support of the facial tissues, and discomfort in eating.

The facts are changing in regard to this disease. For years, we have emphasized controlling plaque. You know—brush and floss your teeth. "But you showed me how to floss my teeth last time!!" Well, get even more used to the lecture, because we have even more information that links gum disease to overall disease. Your body's immune response to plaque in your mouth results in chronic inflammation. That chronic inflammation not only destroys the bone supporting your teeth, it also destroys tissues all over the body. Yes, that's right, all over the body.

But if you think that's all, just hang on here a little longer. While plaque is necessary to start periodontal disease, there are other factors that will worsen it as well as the chronic inflammation in the rest of your body. What is that, pray tell? BAD NUTRITION!!! In fact, nutrition can play a positive or a negative role, depending on how well or poorly you eat. You already know what the bad things are: highly processed food and fast food. Have you ever seen what a McDonald's hamburger looks like four years after it's been cooked? I have one. It looks exactly the same as when I bought it, bun included. How good could that be for you?

The American Heart Association recommends 4-5 servings a day of fresh vegetables and 4-5 servings a day of fresh fruits on a 2000-calorie diet. Yes, that means 8-10 servings (a serving is usually a half cup of a dense fruit or vegetable or a full cup of a leafy vegetable) of delicious fruits and vegetables. That will reduce your risk of heart disease as well as your chances of developing other degenerative diseases, including periodontal disease.

"But I take my vitamins," you say. Sorry, vitamins don't cut it. A multivitamin has, generously, 50-75 nutrients in it; a whole fruit or vegetable—over 12,000 nutrients that have been identified so far. Some studies on vitamins A, C, and E were discontinued because the individuals taking the vitamins were doing worse than those who weren't.

Whole foods is the answer. There are also whole food supplements that you may take to help.

I would recommend that before you brush and floss, have an apple, eat some grapes, dip some carrots in (unprocessed) almond butter. Eat the good foods. They may save more than your teeth.

What supplements do you recommend?

When referring to dental treatment, we usually discuss what we do from the outside. If there's a cavity, we drill it away. If there's periodontal disease, we clean the root surface. If a tooth is missing, we put in a dental implant. All of these treatments are very effective, but they all involve working from the outside. What can we do to build ourselves up from the inside? In 2004 I discovered a nutritional product called Juice Plus. It was recommended to me by a nutritional educator whom I had met several years before. Having been a vegetarian, I know the benefits of fruits and vegetables.

Eating fresh fruits and vegetables is best, but unless we're getting them directly from the farm or from merchants who go directly to the farm, they may not be fresh. How do I know? When I was 16, I worked for a tomato repacking plant in Massachusetts. Here's what I saw: Someone took a large box of tomatoes out of the refrigerator and slowly dumped them onto a conveyor belt. Most of the tomatoes were green. Two women picked out the red ones and packed them in little containers to be delivered to the supermarket. The rest of the tomatoes flowed down the conveyer belt to the end, where they were repacked in a large box. The large box of tomatoes was then put in the refrigerator, waiting to repeat the process a couple of days later. The little containers were wrapped in cellophane with the words "Vine Ripened" printed on the outside.

Do you get 8 to 10 raw servings of fruits and vegetables a day? I don't. Most of the time, I eat in restaurants, so I guarantee you I'm not getting a multitude of vegetables and fruits in my diet.

That's where Juice Plus comes in. Juice Plus is the essence of 17 different fruits and vegetables picked ripe, juiced, dehydrated, and placed in capsules, all within 24 hours of harvest. I started taking Juice Plus because I wanted to have something that was good for me nutritionally and frankly I wasn't seeing that vitamins were doing anything for me. I took Juice Plus for eight months before I recommended it to my patients. During those eight months, I found that my allergies nearly went away. I used to take cortisone shots for allergies once or twice a year, but haven't needed to do so.

Now I would not recommend Juice Plus to you to get rid of your allergies. That isn't the point. The point is that when we don't have adequate amounts of fruits and vegetables, our body does not have the capacity to heal. The body depends upon antioxidants, which get rid of free radicals in our system. Free radicals are charged particles in our systems that cause us to age and to get disease. What impressed me about Juice Plus is that they produce medical scientific research that's done independently in universities and is published in peer-reviewed journals. At this writing, 14 studies on this product have been done. Here's what they confirm:

1. Tremendous numbers of antioxidants introduced into the system.
2. An average reduction of free radicals by 75%.
3. Reduction in constriction of the coronary arteries after a high fat meal.
4. Repair of DNA in a substantial percentage of white blood cells in the elderly population.

5. Reduction in homocysteine levels (which is a predictor of heart disease) in both smokers and non-smokers.

There are studies that are underway, including a study on periodontal disease being done at the University of Wurzberg in Germany, a study on pre-eclampsia, which causes premature births being done in the United States, and a study on hypertension, the preliminary results of which show a dramatic 8-point reduction in the diastolic blood pressure—all of this from good fruits and vegetables in the form of an easy-to-take capsule for about $1.40 a day.

I'm looking forward to hearing the results of the periodontal disease studies, but based on all of this research, I'm recommending it to you. Juice Plus is an absolutely safe and effective product. I hope you'll try it. You can obtain all of the information that you might want by going to my website www.juiceplusdentist.com or talking with any of my office staff.

Your Gums: A Predictor of Heart Disease

IS there a relationship between gum disease and cardiovascular disease? A consensus panel of experts in cardiology and periodontology say, absolutely yes. As a result, members of both professions are making changes in the interest of improving their patients' overall health.

For many years, each of the specialties of the body has been separated. In other words, you see a cardiologist for your heart, a gastroenterologist for your digestive tract, and a periodontist for your gums. These designations were made so that training and expertise could be developed in each area. This gives particular advantage to the patient who has that specialized need.

However, while that separation of specialties makes it convenient for patients to seek the proper practitioner, the body itself is not divided into those arbitrary specialties. The body is the body. We are whole beings.

"But these are my gums," you say. "How can they be related to my heart?" And the other question is, "But I floss my teeth. Isn't that enough?"

Periodontitis, the disease that destroys the bone support for the teeth, is estimated to be present in 30% of the adult population, with severe periodontitis present in 5-15% of the population. Dentists for years have recommended brushing and flossing to remove bacterial plaque to control the onset of gum disease. That recommendation continues, because bacteria are required to initiate the gum disease process. For years, that was the entire story as far as patients and their dentists were concerned. It is not that way any longer. The reason lies in the term, *chronic inflammation.*

Inflammation is the response to bacterial and viral infections and other assaults on the body. The body almost instantly responds to such traumas with acute inflammation, the signs of which are heat, swelling, redness, pain, and loss of function. Acute inflammation allows the needed white blood cells to travel to the site of the assault to begin the healing process. As part of the initial healing process, the cells wall off and eventually engulf and kill the offending bacteria, viruses, or other assaulting agents, also killing the cells that have been infected by those agents. That is acute inflammation, and it is good. The body then creates new cells to complete the healing response.

Chronic inflammation is a continual inflammatory response which occurs in the absence of infection or trauma. Chronic inflammation occurs as a result of obesity, fast foods, smoking, drinking alcohol in excess, refined foods, allergens, environmental toxins, and other agents. In fact, it is chronic inflammation that is believed to be at the center of all chronic disease.

Specifically, periodontitis is caused by dental plaque, yet once the plaque has started the gum lesion, the problem worsens in the presence of chronic inflammation of the body. In addition, the chronic inflammation caused by gum disease may create or increase chronic inflammation in other parts of the body. Examples of diseases associated with chronic inflammation are asthma, diabetes, colitis, nephritis (inflammation of the kidney), some forms of cancer, allergies, and periodontitis and cardiovascular disease.

Several articles in the medical literature report an increased risk of cardiovascular disease in those patients who have periodontitis. Conversely, cardiovascular disease is a risk factor for gum disease and tooth loss. Such a gum risk factor is independent of other traditional risk factors. Periodontitis has been shown to be a risk factor for strokes as well as other forms of cerebrovascular disease. Other risk factors shown to be common between cardiovascular disease and gum disease include diabetes, obesity, high levels of lipids, including cholesterol and triglycerides, and hypertension.

The American Academy of Periodontology has developed a questionnaire to determine your risk of getting periodontitis. Here are some of the questions it includes:

How old are you? Gum disease risk increases as we age.

Do your gums bleed? That is a sign of gum disease. However, if you smoke, you may have gum disease even if your gums do not bleed.

Are your teeth loose? As periodontitis is a chronic inflammatory process, the inflammation results in loss of ligament and bone support for the tooth. Ultimately, it causes loose teeth.

Do you smoke? Smoking is one of the greatest risk factors for gum disease.

Have you seen a dentist in the past two years? Dental hygiene visits allow the removal of dental calculus from the teeth, thus reducing the risk of getting gum disease. Most should see a dentist every 6 months. In the presence of gum disease, 3-month intervals are often recommended.

How often do you floss? Studies have shown that daily flossing reduces the bacteria that cause gum disease.

Do you currently have any of the following health conditions? *Heart disease, osteoporosis, osteopenia, high stress, or diabetes.* If you do, your gum disease risk increases.

Have you ever been told that you have gum problems, gum infection, or gum inflammation? Once any of these occur, continual assessment and monitoring is necessary as gum disease is an ongoing disease in most people.

Have you had any adult teeth extracted due to gum disease? If a tooth was recently lost due to gum disease, your likelihood of losing another tooth increases.

Have any of your family members had gum disease? Research has shown not only a genetic link to gum disease, but also a salivary link. Saliva passed from one family member with gum disease to another may increase that person's risk. People whose parents have gum disease are 6-12 times more likely to have the disease than the general population.

There is a link between nutrition and all chronic degenerative diseases, and one thing can be said for sure; it is whole food nutrition that makes the difference. (You'll see that statement as a running theme in this book.) If it is in a can or in a box, it's not whole food nutrition. The American Heart Association recommends 8-10 servings of fruits and vegetables every day. A serving is ½ cup. Such foods provide the ammunition to battle chronic inflammation, and the better we fight chronic inflammation, the better our opportunity for a healthy life.

For more information on the link between your gums and your heart, please visit the website of the American Academy of Periodontology at www.perio.org.

The Link between Dental Disease and Heart Disease

Dr. Rebecca Hunton
Dr. Lee Sheldon

SEE your dentist to prevent a heart attack? Recently, the research journals and popular press have been pointing to a connection between our oral health and hygiene and our cardiovascular risk. Although there are several mediators, one stands out: periodontal or gum disease. The Journal of Periodontology reported that inflammatory effects from periodontal disease, a chronic bacterial infection of the gums, cause oral bacterial byproducts to enter the bloodstream and trigger the liver to produce substances that increase the risk of heart disease. This is even true in patients who are edentulous (without teeth). Did you know that ill-fitting dentures can create infection and inflammation throughout the mouth that can trigger a systemic effect?

This inflammation is measurable! A substance produced in the body called high-sensitivity C-reactive-protein (HS-CRP) is suspected to play a role in the link between gum disease and heart disease. This test is widely available from traditional labs. Sometimes, CRP is measured in lieu of HS-CRP. The difference? CRP indicates general inflammation while HS-CRP indicates arterial inflammation and increased risk for blood clots. Some studies estimate the HS-CRP is related to dental health over 50 percent of the time! For optimal health, your level should be less than 1. Initially thought to be specific to heart disease, it turns out HS-CRP is a nonspecific marker of inflammation. Inflammation is bad. Data from many studies have shown that long-standing, low levels of inflammation are at the root of most chronic diseases. Think of it this way: HS-CRP is the smoke, and it should put your physician on a search for the fire!

Unfortunately, many adults become lax with their oral health as they age. Frequently, it is because there are no symptoms. We need to think of our mouth as a car, needing frequent oil changes (dental cleanings) and scheduled maintenance (dental exams).

How do you know if you have periodontal disease? The simplest way is to identify periodontal pockets using a periodontal probe. Your dentist and hygienist use such a probe as part of their initial examination as well as your dental cleaning visit. The distance that the probe goes below the gum line is a measure of periodontal damage. A normal measurement is 3 millimeters or less. If you have pockets of 5 or more millimeters, these should be evaluated at every cleaning visit. They will usually improve. If they don't improve, a referral to a periodontist should be considered.

While your physician and dentist are searching for the cause, proper Omega 3 supplementation and the dietary intake of healthy fats and oils has been shown to reduce HS-CRP. In addition, a low-inflammatory diet, weight loss, exercise, and other positive lifestyle changes have an impact on both HS-CRP (inflammation) and other risk factors for chronic disease. If periodontal health is excellent, there are many other causes of elevated HS-CRP that should be investigated. These include vasculitis, cancer, bone infections, inflammatory bowel disease, diabetes, and autoimmune diseases, as well as others.

Remember, we are chasing smoke. Only by finding the fire and addressing it can overall health be improved.

Rebecca Hunton, MD has an integrative medical practice in Viera, FL. She is an expert on the successful application of lifestyle medicine to achieve optimal health and wellness. Dr. Hunton is a preferred provider to members of the NFL Players Association, a member of TEDActive, and most notably, her patients have been featured on the Dr. Oz show to demonstrate successful aging with vitality. Her website is drhunton.com.

Diabetes May Be Improved by Improving Your Periodontal Health

THE statistics on diabetes are staggering. There are nearly two million new diagnoses of diabetes each year. Add that to those who are prediabetic and one of three of us have this problem. And there is more data that may interest you. The health of your gums can influence you diabetes status.

We've known for years that if you're diabetic, you have a greater likelihood of periodontitis, the disease that causes bone loss around your teeth that, if uncontrolled, can result in tooth loss. The more severe the diabetes is, the greater the severity of the periodontitis. In two studies conducted on a diabetic population, periodontal bone loss was from 3 to 11 times greater in that group than in the non-diabetic group.

We have two primary cells involved in bone maintenance: the osteoblast, the cell that forms new bone, and the osteoclast, the cell that removes the old bone. One possible reason for periodontal bone loss in the diabetic is that high blood glucose itself inhibits the production of osteoblasts. High blood glucose levels also hinder the ability of the gums and bone to heal. It doesn't stop there as there is a significant association between periodontitis and your general health. In those diabetics with severe periodontitis, the mortality rate from heart disease was almost 3 times greater, and from kidney disease over 8 times greater, than in the normal population.

However, the reverse may be true as well. Good periodontal control may positively influence your general diabetic condition. Several studies of both Type 1 and Type 2 diabetics have shown a 10% reduction in HbA1c levels (a test that's commonly done to measure the average amount of glucose in the bloodstream over the previous 8-12 week period) by undergoing non-surgical periodontal therapy alone.

So let's look at what that means to you. First, everyone, but particularly the diabetic, needs a thorough assessment of his or her periodontal condition. This includes periodontal probing, x-rays, and an assessment of mobility, bleeding, pus, and other items associated with a full periodontal examination. If periodontitis is diagnosed, the next step is to treat. In most cases, you will have a thorough non-surgical scaling of the teeth below the gum line. This may involve several visits, depending on the severity of the case. This should then be followed with careful monitoring and cleaning, usually every three months. If some areas do not respond to non-surgical therapy because the disease is too far below the gum line, there are a number of surgical approaches that can be used to gain access to the disease and even help replace some or all of the lost bone support.

Periodontal disease is something that must be looked at and treated, not just to save your teeth, but maybe to save your life.

Diabetes and Dental Care

NEARLY every diabetic knows the risks associated with the disease. It's one of the first things that your doctor or nurse talks to you about when the diagnosis is made. There are some dental nuances that affect the diabetic as well.

I've talked about the book *Wheat Belly* in this column. It describes the relationship of wheat to several chronic diseases. I would encourage you, particularly if you are a diabetic, to read it. It proposes a definite negative relationship between the consumption of wheat products and type 2 diabetes. Reading *Wheat Belly* and practicing its philosophy could make a positive impact on reversing your diabetes. That's not a small statement.

Diabetics are certainly more prone to dental diseases as well. Periodontal disease involves the loss of bone support for the teeth. New figures place periodontal disease at 50 percent of the adult population, one of the most prevalent chronic diseases in the United States. It is usually identified by the dentist or hygienist during your dental examination. The bone loss is identified as a "pocket," identified by measuring the distance between the top of the gum line and the underlying attachment to the bone. The deeper the pocket, the more the disease.

In an uncontrolled diabetic, the disease can progress faster than in the normal population. While I don't want to bore you with immunology, there is a lesson to be learned here. Our body's immune system is made up of white blood cells called neutrophils whose sole job is to engulf bacteria and neutralize them. But in diabetes, the neutrophil no longer can sense the bacteria, so the bacteria spread and the pocket gets deeper, leading to loosening of the tooth. This is one reason why diabetics are more prone to generalized infections as well. But if the diabetes is controlled, the neutrophil recovers and can find the bacteria.

While the blood test commonly used is the hemoglobin A1C, which averages your blood sugar control over sixty to ninety days, recent studies indicate that what may be more important is control of "spikes" in your blood sugar. Each spike, which occurs after a high-carbohydrate meal, can cause damage. So for those who feel that you can cheat and then keep your blood sugar low for the next couple of days to make your A1C look better, it just isn't so. That is one reason why your doctor wants you to test your blood sugar throughout the day to be sure that your diabetes is continually under control. That way, your neutrophils are always protecting you from infection.

The good news is that if you are a controlled type 2 diabetic with good periodontal care, you have a good chance of minimizing your periodontal disease and retaining your teeth, and that control will reduce your chance of generalized infections as well.

Bad Breath

WE spend lots of money on products to cover up mouth odor. And whether we're using gum, mints, sprays, or mouthwashes, we are for the most part covering up the cause of halitosis. So let's get to the cause and see if we can make some sense out of this.

What's the main cause of mouth odor? Pure and simple, it is dental disease. Many have the false impression that mouth bacteria are all the same. But of course, that's not true. People with dental disease, and particularly periodontal disease, have different bacteria that cause the bone loss and bleeding associated with the disease. Some people have stinkier bad breath than others, because some types of bacteria smell more than others.

Periodontal disease for the most part can be treated. The question is what treatment is necessary to rid the mouth of bad breath. A thorough periodontal examination is the first requirement, along with appropriate dental x-rays. Periodontal pockets may be indentified. But the pockets are not the cause of the disease, they are the result of the disease. The bacteria and your body's response to the bacteria is the culprit.

We can't identify microscopic bacteria with a clinical examination. Years ago, we tried to culture the bacteria, and had variable results. One reason for that was that we would take the bacteria from the mouth, but by the time the bacteria was received by a laboratory that knows how to look for dental bacteria, much of the bacteria would be altered or dead.

Enter the modern age of periodontal diagnosis. Bacteria have their own unique DNA. The DNA doesn't change whether the bacteria are alive or dead. By merely spitting into a cup and sending that out to a specialized lab that identifies the DNA from oral bacteria, both the type and quantity of your bacteria can be identified. Once we know which bacteria you have, we then can use an antibiotic, if necessary, to help in the elimination of that bacteria. If you happen to have one of the smelly types of bacteria, antibiotic treatment in addition to traditional periodontal treatment can make a nearly instant improvement in your breath.

I won't bore you with the things that you already know you should do and can do better, brushing and flossing. The information that you may not have however is that your tooth surface area is greater in the area between the teeth than on the lip and tongue side of your teeth. So if you're using only a brush, you're getting less than half of the plaque out. The dental hygiene manufacturers have been really good in developing products that help us clean between our teeth better. Those little plastic flossers work better for people who don't have a lot of gum recession. For those who have a lot of gum recession, especially between the teeth, the brushes that go between the teeth may be a better choice. The reason for that is simply that the roots of the teeth are irregular, and a bristle brush is more likely to get into those nooks and crannies.

The tongue itself holds bacteria and food residue. Many people benefit from using tongue cleaners with which you scrape the top of the tongue. What I've found however is that mouth odor from the tongue often originates in the back of the tongue, where the tongue cleaner never reaches. A few drops of a chlorine dioxide mouthwash, such as Clo-Sys, on the back of the tongue can go a long way toward solving the problem.

Could bad breath be caused by something else? Sure. We all know about onion and garlic breath, some of the components of which get right into our blood stream and bathe our lungs and skin in that odor. Could it be a stomach problem or respiratory infection? Sure. But the most likely cause of mouth odor is the mouth. And with a good dental and periodontal examination, and using some of the newer diagnostic and treatment tools, you could be well on your way to solving the problem.

Thin Gums Lead to Sensitive Teeth

WHEN you eat ice cream, do your teeth feel so sensitive that you dare not take another bite? Gum recession can become a gradually worsening problem as we get older. Gum recession occurs because the gum tissue or underlying bone may be thin and have a poor blood supply. While our gum tissue easily stretched over our teeth when we were younger, the tissues get thinner and thinner as we get older and gradually recede.

Recession results in exposure of the root surface. The root surface is softer than tooth enamel. It is much more prone to attacks from acids in the mouth as well as tooth brushing forces. The root continues to wear away, often causing tooth sensitivity.

The treatment for the problem is to move strong gum tissue from another part of the mouth, usually the palate, to the weakened area. This treatment is called a soft tissue graft. If the problem is caught early enough, you can have the gum tissue rebuilt to cover the root surface. Soft tissue grafts are very predictable and are long-lasting. Newer advances in surgical technique allows us to preserve the surface layer of your palate. By harvesting tissue from beneath the surface layer, we can make the healing of the palate much more comfortable. In a small area needing a graft, I like the healing characteristics better by using palatal tissue. And because we can preserve the top layer of the palate, the post-operative discomfort is very mild.

More recently, we do soft tissue grafts using tissues from cadaver sources. This is particularly useful when a patient needs a large graft. Combined with growth factors taken from the platelets in your blood or from animal sources, these grafts are also very predictable and eliminate the need to take donor tissue from the palate.

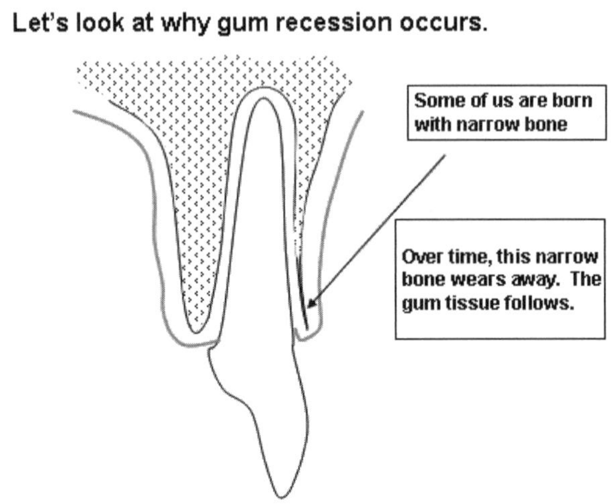

This can present a number of problems. First, the root exposure gives you that "long-in- the-tooth" look. Second, the root exposure often produces tooth sensitivity. Very simply, the top part of our tooth is covered with enamel. Enamel provides a nice thermal layer, like a blanket. But the root doesn't have any enamel, so when we eat cold or sweet things, we feel it right into our roots and sometimes right into our bone. Third, because it is not covered by tough, hard enamel, the root surface itself tends to wear away. This is called "root erosion."

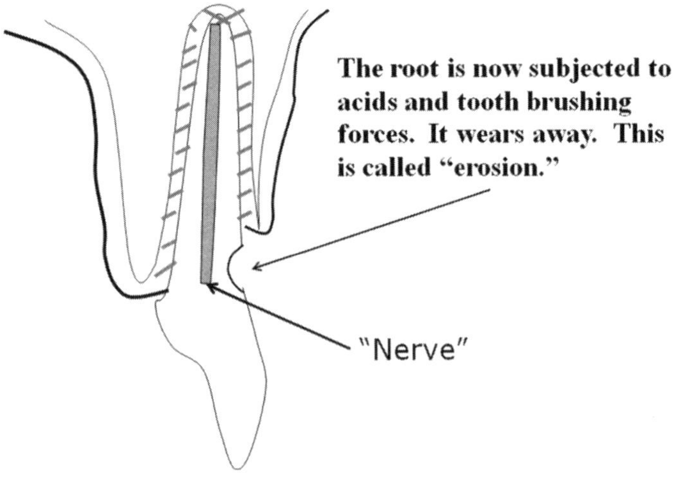

You can feel root erosion. Put your fingernail on your root surface (if it isn't too sensitive) and you may feel that your root is actually gouged. The deeper the gouge, the more sensitive the tooth may be. Moreover, the deeper the gouge, the weaker the tooth may be. I have seen some teeth that have been gouged so deeply that the tooth eventually fractured.

Soft tissue grafting and sometimes even bone grafting will replace the missing bone and gum tissue, often covering the area of root erosion and helping to prevent further recession and erosion.

Case Story

Jacqueline is a physician whose roots were exposed. The roots developed notches (erosion), and she had sensitivity to cold and to sweets. The problem was worsening.

The examination showed thin gums and a likelihood of thin bone. The recommendation that I made to her was to have a procedure done called a "connective tissue graft." This meant that I would be transplanting her own tissue from a layer of tissue under her palate to the area of recession.

(This is not to be confused with the old procedure where we take a "full layer" of tissue from the palate. That procedure produced quite a bit of post-operative discomfort.)

In the connective tissue graft procedure, a piece of tissue is removed from under the top layer of the palate. With the top layer of the palate maintained, this procedure produces very little post-operative discomfort. And so it was with Jacqueline.

"Dr. Sheldon and his wonderful staff made an uncomfortable procedure relatively painless. I was back at work the next day. His knowledge and professionalism is superb and I have no hesitation to return here if I need gum surgery again.
Thanks for a great job!"

Long in the tooth? It can be corrected, reducing sensitivity and improving your smile.

The "Gummy" Smile

AS we age, some of us begin to get the "long in the tooth" look. The reason for that is that the gum tissue and the underlying bone are thin and weak. Over a period of time, the gums recede, exposing the root surface. I have written about several options available to shore up the gums and bone, and in many cases, cover over the exposed root surfaces.

But there is also the opposite problem. Instead of the surrounding gum and bone being thin and receding, the gums and particularly the underlying bone are too thick. That produces what might be called the "short in the tooth" look, or the "gummy smile."

What is the gummy smile? You've seen it. The teeth look short. They've always looked short. When the person smiles, you see more gum than tooth. People are under the misimpression that they are born with short teeth. That is almost never the case. The teeth are actually the correct length. The problem is much of that length is hidden under an overabundance of bone around the tooth, so because the bone is so thick, the gums appear thick and cover much more of the tooth than usual. The remainder of the tooth is hidden beneath that gum and bone tissue. It's like a turtleneck sweater that goes over your chin. Your chin is hidden. It's the same way with the tooth: the neck of the tooth is hidden.

Gummy smiles are not only a cosmetic problem, they can cause other problems as well. If, for example, you get a cavity between the teeth, the cavity is much more difficult to treat because the decay is buried beneath the excess bone and gum tissue. You may get bleeding and a periodontal pocket as a result because the filling is intruding into the space occupied by the gum and bone.

The good news is that the gummy smile and overabundant gum and bone tissue can be treated, and while the treatment for this problem is surgical in nature, the healing after the surgery is comfortable and the results are permanent.

Here's what is done: The periodontist will lift the gum tissue away from the teeth and bone and then sculpt the bone around those teeth into the proper shape. The gum tissue is then returned to place. Because the underlying bone is no longer propping up the gum tissue, the gum can now rest in the proper relationship with the tooth. The result is front teeth that are the correct length, taller than they are wide. The result is back teeth are the correct length, allowing for crowns to be placed in their proper position, making them less likely to fall off or cause tissue irritation.

So when you smile, if you see short teeth, rest assured that those teeth are not really short. The rest of those teeth are hidden, and with just the right surgical procedure, your teeth can look totally normal.

Some Gum Problems Are not really a Disease, but Need to Be Treated

THERE are a host of other periodontal problems which are not really a disease. Here are the periodontal problems that, while not diseases, still threaten the tooth and need to be recognized and addressed. Some have already been mentioned in previous chapters. They are being repeated now for completeness.

Recession is the exposure of the root surface caused by the retraction of the soft tissue. Recession is most often caused by the wearing away of a thin layer of bone under the gum line, which occurs as we get older. The exposure of the root surface to the outside can be dangerous because the roots are softer than the enamel of the tooth. They are therefore prone to developing wear, grooves, and sensitivity. They can get so worn that the teeth break. Recession is usually a genetic problem, as the width of the bone is literally narrower than the tooth itself. In other words, you have a size 8 tooth fitting into a size 2 bone. The recession can sometimes worsen with overzealous tooth brushing.

Altered Passive Eruption is just the opposite. Here you have too much gum and bone. The tooth appears short. It really isn't. It's just hiding under overabundant gum tissue. When it happens on the front teeth, they appear squat. When it occurs on the back teeth, it involves more than the appearance. The problem is cavities. Cavities that would ordinarily be easy to reach are now buried under gum tissue. It makes doing a filling very difficult for the dentist and makes home care very difficult as well. Sometimes the filling needs to be placed so deeply that the gums bleed, and there's soreness when you chew.

The treatment for altered passive eruption is surgical exposure of the tooth by removing the excess gum and bone. It sounds a little rough, but these surgical procedures are some of the easiest for our patients to handle.

Normal Bone

The primary reason you have a gummy smile or short teeth has nothing to do with the teeth themselves.

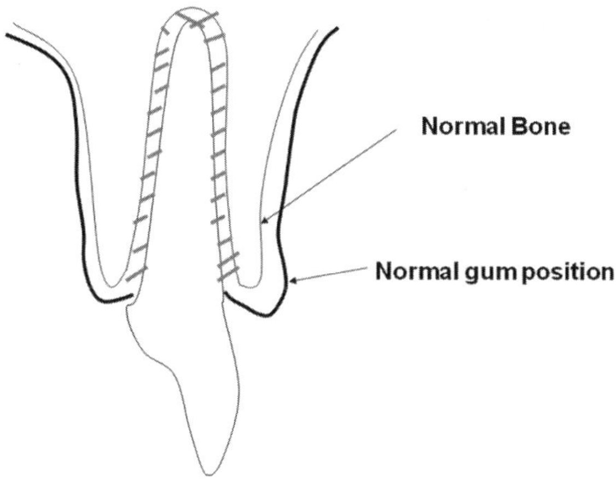

Thick Bone

It more often has to do with the thickness of the underlying bone.

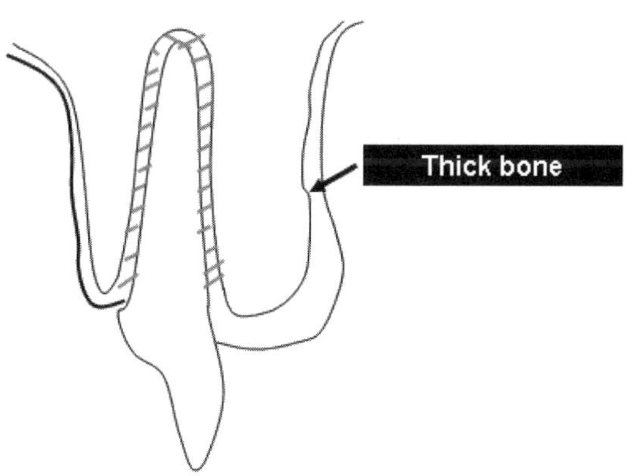

Case Story

As we age, we sometimes acquire that long-in-the-tooth-look. Sherry had exactly that, with gums receding and the roots showing. She was embarrassed to smile. In another part of her mouth, her teeth were very short and she had a gummy smile. To have long teeth in one area and short teeth in another is an unusual combination, but the fact is that the short teeth can be made longer and the long teeth can be made shorter through appropriate periodontal plastic surgery procedures. Here's what Sherry says:

"My dentist referred me to Dr. Sheldon to have a soft tissue graft. Upon consultation, Dr. Sheldon advised me that my teeth were too short and by having crown lengthening of my upper teeth, I would have much better smile.

After I agreed to proceed with all of the above (in one sitting!!), I had a great deal of apprehension, and decided I had lost whatever common sense I might have possessed. The staff at Dr. Sheldon's office was helpful and caring and made me feel at ease.

The pre-op instructions were clear and easy to follow. The surgery went amazingly well and I had no problems whatsoever. The healing process was faster than I imagined and in no time at all, I had the promised smile. There was no part of the procedure or healing that was anywhere near as bad as I expected.

Imagine how pleased I am after 50-something years of having short teeth, I am now not long in the tooth, but I am told I have a wonderful smile! Thanks to Dr. Sheldon and his great staff!"

– Sherry R.

Why Non-surgical Treatment Is Best for Some Problems

WHEN do you do non-surgical treatment, and when do you do surgical treatment? I must say that this is a controversy. As I write this, I have just seen a nice woman who wanted to get a third opinion. She wouldn't tell me anything about the first two opinions, nor would she tell me what treatment she had undergone. That's a difficult game for me to play, but I decided to play anyway. (Besides that, my assistant told me what had happened before to this patient, as the patient was willing to tell her but unwilling to tell me. Do you really think that our staff doesn't communicate with the doctor? Who do you think pays them? *Don't tell him* is not a part of the language we speak in our office, and for good reason. If I don't know something about you, I don't know how to evaluate your response to whatever you don't want me to know. If you've had periodontal treatment with another periodontist, that's absolutely fine. I need to know your response to that treatment before I can make appropriate recommendations for treatment in our office.)

Anyway, I did the full periodontal examination and looked at the x-rays that had been taken by someone else. What I saw in the examination looked much better than what I saw in the x-rays. So, even without my beautiful, loyal, skilled assistant, I already knew that this woman had received some treatment before she saw me. So what I saw was a healing state. The patient was doing better now. That's good! The previous periodontist did a great job.

Now here's her story. She saw a periodontist who recommended doing a non-surgical procedure first to see how well things would heal before deciding on surgery. The periodontist saw an improved condition, but there were still some periodontal pockets. He decided that the best way to treat this would be to surgically eliminate the pockets. That's a very common approach. She saw a second periodontist who recommended much the same, but surgical treatment of fewer teeth. So she sought me for a third opinion. She obviously didn't want surgery or she would have stopped at opinion 1 or opinion 2. She showed good evidence of healing following the treatment from the first periodontist. So the question would be, is there any harm in waiting to see if the response might get even better? The answer is a clear NO. There absolutely is no harm done. I can see her every three months for a cleaning. She can perform good home care, which, by the way, was already excellent, and I can see whether she heals further. She may be able to maintain things exactly as is or improve without my so much as touching her with a scalpel. Should things start to go downhill again, that would mean surgical treatment is necessary, either to remove bacterial deposits below the gum line or to help the patient grow new bone attachment for the tooth. But we can often wait and monitor the patient every three months before we have to make such a decision.

Therefore, my rule #1 for treatment of chronic periodontitis is: if a patient shows substantial healing following non-surgical therapy, stop and observe.

It may continue to get better. If it doesn't get better, I can always do surgery later on. In the meantime, just get a good cleaning every 3 months or so, and let's observe the progress of the periodontal pockets. This isn't just my idea. There are reams of literature to support this concept.

Now let's go back a step. What is good, non-surgical therapy and where does it apply? If a patient has lost bone support and has pockets with calculus and plaque, he or she is a candidate for non-surgical therapy. That is a very plain rule. The purpose of non-surgical therapy is to get as much of the calculus and plaque out of the pocket as possible so that the gums and bone will heal.

Non-surgical therapy depends upon three things:

1. the skill of the therapist
2. the availability of a wide variety of sharp instruments that can get into any nook or cranny that's present in the pocket

3. the ability to find the plaque and calculus

Number 3 has improved. Up until now, we relied upon "feeling" the calculus on the root surface with the dental instruments that we use. We know that we can't feel calculus very well any more than you can feel your way around a dark room in a strange house. The literature proves that beyond 4 mm, we can't clean a pocket very well at all by feel.

That's all changed with the dental endoscope. The endoscope is a tiny camera that is small enough to be placed in the pocket. We can now see the calculus, and when we can see the calculus, we can get it out. The literature shows that as well. One reason that we do periodontal surgery is so that we can see the calculus to get it out. Even then, we can't see very well between teeth and on the backsides of teeth during surgery. The endoscope helps us look between teeth, between roots, around corners. It's just an amazing device. And while it is a relatively rarely found instrument (there are only 200 in the United States), we find it invaluable in detecting and removing calculus. We've had our endoscope for over ten years. I don't think we'd ever go back to not using it in moderate and severe periodontitis cases. **It is helping our patients stay out of surgery.** I haven't met a person yet who would rather have surgery. Are you an exception?

Why Surgical Treatment Is Best for Some Problems

WHY do you need surgery? That's a good question. Let's not get carried away. This is not a life or death situation. These are your teeth. You'll survive without teeth. I quickly state, however, that you'll likely live a shorter life without teeth. There's data to support that. So when you are considering surgery to help save your teeth, why would you do it?

Here are the reasons:

1. The periodontist needs to see below the gum line to remove embedded calculus on the root surface.
2. The tooth is too short or a cavity or crack in the tooth is too deep below the gum line to be properly restored.
3. You have a good chance of re-growing some of the lost bone and lost ligament with surgical treatment.
4. You need to replace weak and deteriorated gum tissue with healthy gum tissue.
5. You need a correction to cover exposed roots.
6. You want to make your cosmetically short teeth longer and get rid of the "gummy smile."
7. You need to extract a bad tooth because the disease from the bad tooth is spreading to the neighboring tooth.
8. You need to replace a missing tooth or a badly damaged tooth with a dental implant.

If there is a non-surgical option available, explore it. If not, or if non-surgical treatment doesn't offer a good prognosis, you might as well jump to the next step. **It is far more predictable to do surgical treatment when the teeth and root surfaces are clean than to wait for an infection to occur.**

What Is "Crown Lengthening and Root Reshaping?"

CROWN lengthening! What a confusing term! First of all, there are so many definitions of crown. If we don't know the definitions of crown, how would we know what "crown lengthening" is? So let's do what we should always do when we don't understand something—define our terms or look them up in a good dictionary. For now, I'll give you the definitions, and there are three worth noting in dentistry.

Crown def. 1: the part of the tooth that's above the gum line. In other words, this is the part of the tooth that you can see. It's called the *clinical crown.*

Crown def. 2: the part of the tooth that's covered with enamel. It's called the *anatomic crown.* So if part of the enamel is under the gum line, it means that the anatomic crown is longer than the clinical crown. That's another definition for altered passive eruption, which is covered in a previous chapter.

Crown def. 3: an artificial covering for a tooth that has broken down. It is made out of a variety of materials, but is usually gold and porcelain or porcelain alone. It's often called a *cap.*

There are times when I'll see a patient for a crown lengthening consultation, and the damage to the tooth is so extensive that I would have to remove a great deal of bone, resulting in a weaker tooth or a gum line that would be esthetically changed. If that's the case, I'll recommend preserving the bone by extracting the tooth and placing a titanium metal post in the bone called a dental implant. Your dentist then uses the dental implant to support the new crown (cap).

Here's why crown lengthening is important. Let's assume that a tooth fractures below the gum line. Your dentist would have to bury the crown even deeper below the gum line, thereby **causing permanent gum bleeding and possibly pain.** If a tooth is too short, the crown is likely to fall off.

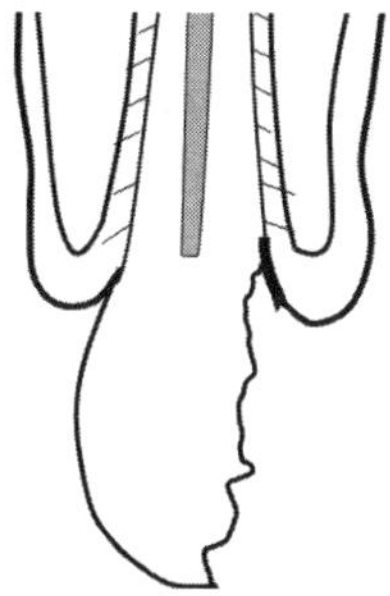

A crown restoration would need to be buried below the gum line, causing permanent gum pain.

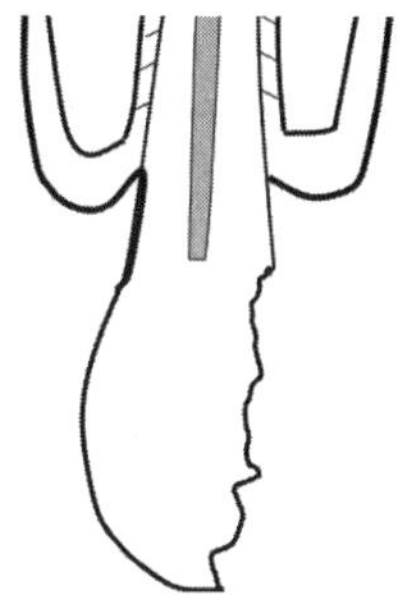

After crown lengthening

The procedure that we do to remedy this problem is called "crown lengthening" or crown extension. We're making the *clinical crown* (the part of the tooth that shows) longer so that the *crown restoration* will fit correctly. It should really be called "tooth lengthening" to avoid all of the confusion with the word, *crown.*

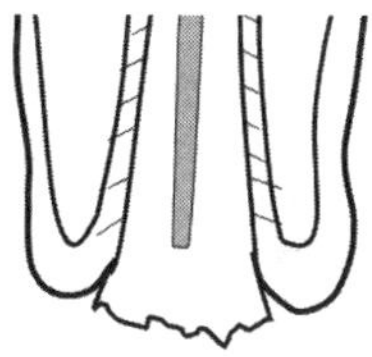

A crown on a tooth that is this badly fractured would fall off.

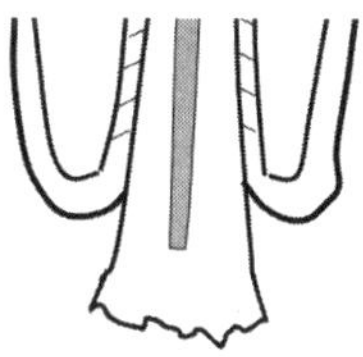

After crown lengthening

The next step may be a procedure called "root reshaping." Root reshaping allows the periodontist to shape the tooth correctly below the gum line, making the crown restoration easier for the general dentist and the patient. For some, it means less gum and bone removal and therefore a stronger tooth.

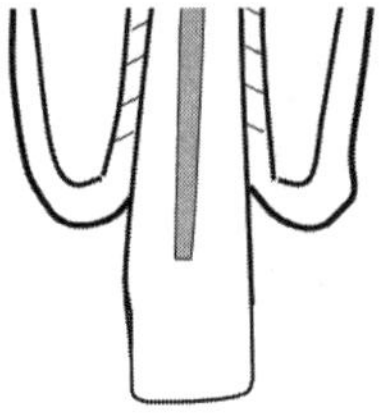

After root reshaping

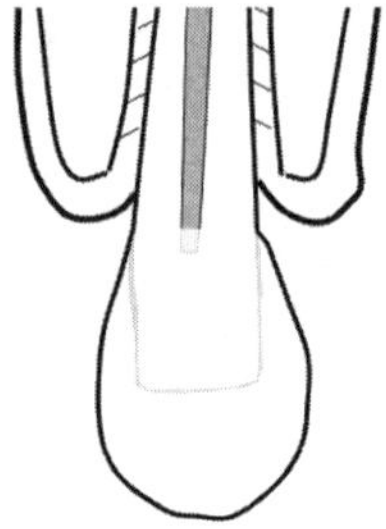

New, properly fitting crown

If too much bone needs to be removed or if the tooth is too weak to provide long-term success, a better choice may be a dental implant. A dental implant will allow you to keep most, if not all, of your bone. Therefore, some judgment is involved. How long must the tooth be to retain a crown? How much bone support will need to be removed to create that length? How much will that alter the gum line and what will it look like? Will a dental implant create more long-term stability?

Answering these questions before doing major treatment will help ensure that your investment in that tooth is a wise one.

Case Story

At times there is a choice to make. Do we save teeth or do we replace them with dental implants? The key is to save the teeth that can be saved and to replace the teeth that need to be replaced early, before dental implant supporting bone is gone. If dental implant supporting bone recedes too much, there can be aesthetic problems. Here is Dona's story:

"Two years ago I arrived at Dr. Sheldon's Melbourne office seeking a second opinion with regard to my seriously progressive

periodontal disease. I had been told that my case was so advanced that I would have to settle for a partial plate or possibly dentures. My family dentist recommended that before making any decision, I should seek the opinion of Dr. Lee Sheldon. The recommendation changed my life.

Today I have four perfect implants, four crowns, no periodontal disease whatsoever, and a simply beautiful smile. This is particularly important to me because I am a flight attendant. My smile is the first thing my passengers notice about me and now I can greet my guests with total self-confidence.

Last but not least, I would like to compliment Dr. Sheldon, himself, for caring about each and every patient the way he does. For him, making people happy is not just a vocation; it is an avocation. You can see this in the way he hand selects his wonderful staff. From the moment you are greeted at the front desk right to the time of surgery and follow-up cleaning visits, you know that Dr. Sheldon has personally chosen all of these caring employees for their compassion and knowledge. As you sit in the lounge area and read this letter, know that you are in the best possible hands. Know that these people truly care about you and know that you will soon be smiling as you have never smiled before. Sincerely with thanks, Dona L."

TOOTH DECAY AND RESTORATIVE SOLUTIONS

My Teeth Continue to Have Cavities

YOU thought the days of cavities were over when you were a kid. But what happens as we get older? We get cavities again—one of those miracles of aging gracefully.

The problem with cavities in an adult is that they happen in the most inaccessible areas, usually on the exposed root at the gum line. Those cavities are difficult to treat. There is no dentist who enjoys treating those cavities, and they tend to recur because the problem that caused the cavities remains.

What's the problem? When we were young our saliva had a neutral pH. That means the mouth generally wasn't acidic. Our saliva glands don't work as well as they used to and many of the medications that are taken to treat chronic diseases cause dry mouth. Dry mouths are acidic. People with dry mouths can get a lot of cavities.

Here's what you can do about it: 1) Talk with your doctor and determine whether you might be able to withdraw from some of those medications. 2) Reduce the sugar in your diet. Sugar comes in many forms. Processed food has sugar. Candies, cakes, sweets? You know them all. Sugar increases the incidence of decay. 3) Measure the acid level of your mouth. Your dentist may be able to help you with that, or you can go to the drugstore and buy nitrazine test paper. Put a small piece of this acid-detecting paper in your mouth. Once the paper is wet, it will turn a certain color and you can measure the color of the paper against a color chart and determine your pH (acid level). It should be a pH of 7.

Here are some new approaches: One is xylitol. Xylitol is a sugar. You can buy it in any health food store. Xylitol has been shown to remineralize decaying tooth structure. The second is a rinse which neutralizes the pH. If you don't produce enough saliva, you can buy a rinse that does. Your dentist or your pharmacist will recommend one to you. You are looking for a rinse with a pH of 7.0 or as close to that as possible. A simple home remedy is to use baking soda rinses. Their pH is higher than 7.0, but will neutralize acids very fast. Take a tablespoon of baking soda, mix it in 8 ounces of water, and just rinse with a mouthful of it and spit out. Most only need do this 3 or 4 times a day. The third is to eat more raw vegetables. The fourth is to use the new calcium phosphate products which assist in the remineralization of enamel. You can look them up on the internet.

And now there is a rinse that addresses all of the causes of dental decay. The rinse is called Cari-Free. It is a little pricey, but with the expense of dental care, the cost of the rinse may well be worth it.

With diligence to detail, you can reverse the trend of tooth decay in your own mouth and save money, discomfort, and tooth loss.

Your Dry Mouth Could Be Killing Your Teeth

WHAT do over five hundred medications have in common? The medications treat various chronic problems all over the body. But they can create major problems for your teeth. Why? Because these medications reduce saliva production. They cause dry mouth.

Saliva just doesn't make our mouths wet; it protects our teeth from bacterial attack. Good, healthy saliva acts as a buffer to neutralize acidic foods. No saliva? Your mouth's acid level increases. The acid-loving bacteria in your mouth have a field day. Our teeth decay, and this decay is not just a nuisance repaired by a simple filling. It can dissolve exposed roots. Sometimes it happens so fast that nothing can be done to save the tooth, and it needs to be extracted.

Dry mouth can occur as a result of some chronic diseases such as Sjogren's syndrome. It can occur following radiation therapy to the head and mouth region as well as after chemotherapy.

So what's the solution? If you are taking medications that are causing dry mouth, one thing you can do is to ask your physician if there is an alternative medication. Barring that, you need to do your best to keep the mouth moist and the acid reduced. A constant water bottle by your side is one solution. But even then, there is no assurance that the mouth acids will be neutralized. I have my patients rinse with baking soda rinses up to four times a day. Make a solution of 1 tablespoon of baking soda to 8 ounces of water. Rinse for 1 minute and spit. The 8 ounces of water should last the full day.

There are artificial salivas that you can purchase from your pharmacy as well.

There is a natural sugar that actually can reverse tooth decay: xylitol.

Xylitol comes as a straight granulated sugar. I recommend, however, that you purchase xylitol mints or xylitol gum. Make sure that the mints or gum are 100-percent xylitol with no other added sugars. Dissolve 5 mints a day or chew 5 pieces of gum a day spread throughout the day. You can find xylitol in health food stores and many dental offices.

An excellent rinse to help prevent dental decay is Cari-Free. It combines an acid modifier, xylitol, and modifies the bacterial imbalance in the mouth. It can be ordered online at carefree.com

Finally, increase the frequency of your dental examinations.

Dry mouth can be devastating to your teeth. It requires a change in how you treat your mouth even if you haven't had a decay problem in the past. Aggressive preventive care can go a long way in reducing your dental expenses as well as your chance of tooth loss.

It's Not Too Late for Cosmetic Dentistry.

AT the risk of sounding vain, I'm about to do a procedure that I've said for years that I "don't need." That is cosmetic dentistry.

Yes, I know that many know me and are accustomed to my teeth. They are in great shape, almost no dental work in my mouth. Just got lucky, I guess. But you also know that I have spaces between my teeth. I always did. Over the years, the spaces widened in one area just a bit. When I saw myself in a picture taken from the left side, there was a pretty wide gap between two of my teeth. I went to my friend who had recommended cosmetic dentistry to fill all the gaps between my teeth. He even did a cosmetic workup, where through the magic of computer imagery, I was able to see what I would look like with the spaces filled. I looked at the image and told him to just narrow the gap between the two most "distinctive" teeth. He put some tooth-colored filling material there, and it did the trick.

One of the dentists in my office, Dr. Jennifer Chace, approached me earlier this year. She said, "How about a cosmetic workup?" I said that I'd gone that route already and declined. She said, "How about if we do it directly on you?" Meaning, how about if you see in your own mouth what you would look like? In a weak moment, I said okay.

She took molds of my mouth and asked the dental laboratory to fill in the spaces on the model and reshape the teeth. I saw the restored model of my teeth. My gaps were gone. She then had a mold made of the restored teeth. She put tooth-colored filling material in the mold, put the mold in mouth, and ten minutes later, I was able to smile and see what my teeth could look like in my own mouth. I smiled, and I couldn't believe the difference. Each of my staff members came in to see the result. They all loved it. (You can see the before and after on this page.) Of course, this was only a temporary result. The filling material was easily flicked off, but the fact is that I could see what I *could* look like, and even though I am sixty-two years old, I decided right then to do the procedure.

I will be doing veneers on ten of my top teeth. Why ten? Because those are the teeth that show when I smile. For the result to look consistent, you need to include every tooth in the smile.

For those of you who have been thinking about it at all, ask your dentist for a cosmetic workup. Your dentist can do what Dr. Chace is doing for me. And who knows? Maybe more of us will rejuvenate our smiles together.

Tooth Whitening

Matthew E. Sheldon, DMD

ARE your teeth more yellow than they used to be? Have you tried over-the-counter whitening products such as whitening toothpastes, strips, mouthwashes, and gels? Do you find that they just don't do the trick? There is a safe and effective way to get your teeth multiple shades whiter at the dentist. It is called intraoral whitening.

Whitening, also commonly known as bleaching, has been used in dental offices for many years. The most common active ingredient used for bleaching is hydrogen peroxide. The hydrogen peroxide reacts with the darker molecules in your teeth, the browns and yellows, and lightens them. The result is a whiter, brighter smile.

There are two types of discolorations on teeth: intrinsic and extrinsic stains. Intrinsic stains are stains on the inside of the tooth. Aging, injury to the tooth, fluorosis, and exposure to antibiotics while your teeth were developing can cause intrinsic stains. Extrinsic stains are discolorations on the tooth surface. This can be caused by tobacco, soda, red wine, tea, coffee, and poor oral hygiene. Whitening agents can reduce stains caused by both types of discoloration, but the easier to remove are the extrinsic stains.

There are a few ways to whiten your teeth. The first is in-office whitening. In-office whitening uses high concentration hydrogen peroxide and a special light to help accelerate whitening. Your dentist will first place a barrier over your gums for protection, paint on the whitening agent, and then use the special light on your teeth for a period of up to one hour. Lights are typically within the blue spectrum, as blue light is thought to be able to enhance the effect of the hydrogen peroxide. There are ongoing studies to determine if the light helps accelerate whitening or if it's the action of the high concentration hydrogen peroxide alone that allows your teeth to be multiple shades whiter in about an hour. In-office whitening is the quickest way to get your teeth whiter, but due to the high concentration of hydrogen peroxide, your teeth may temporarily become sensitive. This method is popular for people looking for last-minute whitening for a big event, like a wedding, reunion, etc.

Another way to whiten teeth is dentist-prescribed, at-home whitening. Your dentist will take impressions of your mouth, fabricate custom whitening trays on the models developed from the impressions, and give you whitening gel to use at home. The whitening gels come in different concentrations based on the strength appropriate for you. We take special care to ensure excess gel doesn't spill over onto your gums by making precise custom trays to carry the gel to your teeth only. Common at-home whitening systems are used thirty minutes per day for up to two weeks. This is a very popular method allowing you the freedom of doing it yourself at home, while being able to use prescription strength whitening agents.

The last way to whiten your teeth is using the over-the-counter methods. You will see an aisle full of these at the drugstore. There are strips, trays, mouthwashes, toothpastes, and pens. All of these methods have a lower concentration of whitening agent than what your dentist can prescribe, taking longer or not ever reaching your desired results. The strips and the trays are not custom-fit to your mouth. The mouthwashes and toothpastes can remove some surface stains but nothing more than you would see after a dental cleaning. For the hydrogen peroxide to work, it needs the proper amount of time to sit on your teeth. That's why you may be disappointed with most over-the-counter products.

Whitening does not work on most dental restorations. Hydrogen peroxide is meant to work on your natural tooth structure. So if some of your front teeth have fillings or crowns, the whitening will not have an effect on those restorations. This will leave you with uneven whitening throughout your mouth. Your dentist will be able to tell you which method of whitening will give you your desired results.

Digital Impressions: The Goop Is Gone

Matthew E. Sheldon, DMD

FINAL impressions—most of us have had them taken at one time or another for a number of reasons. That is the impression we take so we have a model of your mouth. We take them when you need a crown, bridge, veneer, inlay, onlay, implant abutment, implant crown or bridge, and braces. The material that is used to take this final impression starts out runny. The dentist places it in a tray and puts it in your mouth and lets it set for up to seven minutes. The impression material gets very rigid, and then the dentist pulls it out of your mouth. Hopefully, we captured everything we wanted to. If not, it's time to start the process all over again. If you have an active gag reflex, an impression is no picnic. Once we have a good impression, the laboratory then pours a liquid dental stone into it, lets the stone set, and removes the stone model from the impression. The stone model is now a replicate of your mouth. Now we and the laboratory, working together, create your restoration or design your braces. A lot of dental offices still use this method, and we sometimes need to as well.

But there is a more effective, more accurate, and kinder way to take that final impression using digital and computer electronics. Instead of the goop, there is a wand with a tiny camera on it that takes thousands of pictures of your mouth and teeth. It captures all the same areas that are captured with the goop. This benefits you in a number of ways. It's precise, you can take breaks in the middle of the impression if you need to, and there's no mess.

We don't have to pour a model either. Instead the pictures are sent over the Internet to our digital impression provider, where a special machine carves out a model of your mouth. This makes everything as accurate as possible. The dentist can analyze the model of your mouth from every angle on a wide-screen computer monitor. This gives the dentist one last chance to make any corrections to your teeth before the model is sent to the lab for your final restoration. The result with the digital way is a more accurate, better fitting crown, bridge, veneer, etc. As a dentist, I work in the mouth every day and look at teeth upside-down and backwards in mirrors, peeking around lips, cheeks, and tongues. The digital impression gives the dentist a chance to look at the teeth that they worked on, zoomed in and from any angle. It provides the chance to make the teeth more beautiful and virtually eliminates the need for any remakes.

For patients doing Invisalign or similar orthodontic treatment, the iTero digital scanner is the perfect complement. A big bonus for the patient is the Invisalign Outcome Simulator, which helps you visualize your new smile in minutes before even beginning treatment. Your clear Invisalign aligners are ready twice as fast as those done with traditional impressions, so treatment starts that much faster, and the improved accuracy of the iTero digital scanner means the fit of your aligners is that much better.

The experiences my patients and I have had using this technology have been tremendous. The crowns, bridges, veneers, inlays, onlays, implant custom abutments, implant crowns and bridges, and Invisalign clear braces that come back from the laboratory are as close to perfect as we can get. The fit and adjustments needed to make the bite perfect are minimal. That means there is less adjustment time and shorter office visits. In the hundreds of scans we have done at the office, I have yet to have a patient tell me they preferred the other way to take an impression. So yes, there is a way to eliminate the goop and produce a quicker, more accurate result in the process.

Selecting the Correct Crown

Matthew E. Sheldon, DMD

IN the profession of dentistry, diagnosis and treatment planning are as important as the treatment itself. Over the years, my patients have told me that they appreciate being included in the decision-making process for their treatment. As a result, I am continuously thinking of options to suit my patients' functional, esthetic and financial needs. In the practice of general dentistry, one treatment that has numerous options is the crown.

The crown, commonly known as a *cap,* is a restoration that completely encircles and protects a natural tooth or dental implant post. The crown is used to restore a natural tooth for several reasons: a large cavity is too large to hold a filling, a tooth is fractured, an existing filling needs to be replaced because of leakage, a root canal treated tooth needs to be restored, or a space between teeth needs to be closed.

There are three fundamental types of crowns; all-metal, porcelain-fused-to-metal, and all-ceramic. In the past, the 'gold standard' for molar teeth that needed crowns was, well, gold. Owing to its compatibility and strength, gold is very durable and long lasting. Additionally, it wears similarly to your natural teeth and adapts well to the margins that your dentist creates when preparing your tooth. Out of all the dental materials, gold needs the least amount of bulk for its strength. What does that mean for you, the patient? Gold requires less removal of the good or healthy part of your tooth in order to support the restoration. There are two drawbacks to the gold crown, the price of gold and the cosmetics of gold.

Porcelain-fused-to-metal crowns, or PFMs, are another great option for both back and front teeth. PFMs are exactly what they sound like, metal (usually a gold alloy) on the inside and porcelain on the outside. This combination provides the strength of metal and the esthetics of porcelain. The PFM provides excellent strength but the porcelain can chip exposing the metal underneath. This is seen especially in patients who grind their teeth. Due to the fact that the base of the crown is metal, a dark line may appear at the base of the crown where it joins the porcelain, particularly at the gum line. You should discuss esthetic expectations with your dentist prior to doing any crown restoration. For example, if a patient presents signs of excessive grinding, the dentist may choose to use more metal in the chewing surface of the crown rather than a porcelain chewing surface. Such treatment expectations need to be addressed in advance of the final restoration. We don't want any surprises.

All-ceramic crowns, once limited to the front teeth due to their fragility, are now placed throughout the mouth. The high demand for esthetics coupled with scientific research has produced a beautiful-appearing crown that can be used anywhere in the mouth. There are many types of all-ceramic crowns and, without getting too specific, they are: all-porcelain, porcelain-fused-to-zirconia, and all-zirconia. When comparing porcelain to zirconia, porcelain has a higher esthetic quality but is not nearly as strong. If you are looking for a more natural-looking crown that can still provide strength and durability, you may choose a porcelain-fused-to-zirconia crown. The down side to this type of crown is that it requires a large bulk of material for strength and therefore more tooth structure must be removed in the tooth preparation process. Alternatively, an all-zirconia crown, while strong, lacks the esthetic quality of porcelain. If esthetics is not a top priority, this would be a good option for a patient that is a heavy grinder. Again, keeping an open-dialogue with your dentist is important. He or she will be able to choose the ceramic crown that best suits your needs.

When deciding what type of crown is best for you, here are some important questions to ask:

- Are you a grinder?
- Do you have any known metal allergies?
- Is esthetics a top priority?
- Are you willing to sacrifice durability for your esthetic demands?

There are a number of materials with which a crown can be constructed and being informed can help you and your dentist choose the best material for you.

Onlays

Matthew E. Sheldon, DMD

MANY patients have been through the following scenario. You get a cavity on a back tooth and your dentist removes the cavity and places a filling on the tooth. Then the filling wears away or you get a new cavity on that tooth and your dentist either redoes the filling or the cavity is so large that it requires a more permanent restoration, such as a crown. In some cases, the crown doesn't have to be the next step, and you may be able to have an onlay.

Let's quickly review our definition of a dental crown. It is a restoration made out of porcelain, zirconia, or gold that is placed over the entire tooth. Your dentist removes part of the tooth all the way around to accommodate this restoration and protect your tooth from further injury. If a crown needs to be replaced, the only option is a new crown. Your tooth can only be recrowned a limited number of times before your dentist runs out of healthy tooth structure to support any restoration.

But there is a more conservative answer that preserves more tooth structure: the onlay. The onlay is like a dental crown, but it doesn't completely cover the tooth. Your dentist removes only the unhealthy portion of the tooth and replaces it with the same materials as a crown. Because only part of the tooth is being replaced, it fits on your tooth like a puzzle piece. If there is ever a need for a new restoration, you have more of your own tooth to rely on. This gives you and your dentist more predictable options in the future.

To find out if you qualify for an onlay, your dentist will first need to diagnose the problem with the tooth. He or she will look for cavities, cracks, and missing tooth structure on your tooth through x-ray and visual diagnosis. Then if it's determined that you have enough healthy tooth to support a restoration that partially covers your tooth, your dentist may recommend an onlay.

An onlay takes two dental visits to complete. Your tooth will be numbed and then prepared for an onlay. Depending on your dentist, a digital impression or a conventional impression is taken of the prepared tooth. A temporary restoration is made at the end of the first visit. Then your dentist and the laboratory design the onlay for proper color, shape, and bite. The second visit is to permanently deliver your new onlay. You and your dentist will evaluate the color, shape, and bite before permanently bonding it into place.

Onlays can be made of porcelain or gold. Onlays protect teeth and are a great option for you when indicated.

Veneers: Esthetically Changing the Shape and/or Color of Your Teeth

Matthew E. Sheldon, DMD

IN a previous chapter, we talked about what whitening can do for your smile, but what if your teeth won't get white enough, or you don't like the shape of your teeth? Dental veneers are the answer for healthy teeth that are not esthetically pleasing to the patient.

Dental veneers have become popular over the years due to increased patient demand for cosmetic dentistry. They have been featured on the popular extreme makeover shows. Most patients have heard about veneers, but what are they, and could you be a candidate?

Veneers are custom-made shells of tooth-colored material designed to cover the front surface of your teeth to improve their appearance. They can be used on healthy teeth that are discolored, chipped, uneven, worn down, or irregularly shaped, or to close gaps between teeth. The veneers can be made wafer-thin, meaning that only a minimal amount of healthy tooth structure needs to be removed to create an esthetic veneer.

To find out if veneers are the best treatment option, you and your dentist will first need to discuss what you would like improved and your expectations. Impressions of your existing teeth should be taken prior to preparing your teeth for veneers. The models of your teeth made from these impressions serve many functions. Your dentist can improve your chipped teeth on the models by placing tooth-colored wax on each of the teeth. This is called a "wax-up." The wax-up gives you a visualization of what is necessary to get to your desired results. Both you and your dentist can see what can be achieved, and both of you have the chance to critique and change the wax-up as desired before you ever start treating the teeth themselves.

Once a treatment plan is developed, the next step is tooth preparation. Oftentimes, dental anesthesia is not needed due to the minimal amounts of tooth structure that is removed. Once your dentist is satisfied with your tooth preparations, he or she will take a final impression. You will leave the office with temporary veneers. Although these won't be as beautiful as the final restorations, they do give you the opportunity to assess the shape and length of what the final veneers will look like. We can adjust your temporaries to your liking, and when you and your dentist are agreed, a photo and a model of the adjusted temporaries is also sent to the laboratory. The lab then creates your final veneers based upon those temporaries.

The next appointment will be to deliver your veneers. The temporaries will be removed, the teeth receiving the veneers will be cleaned, and the permanent veneers will be tried-in with temporary cement. This gives you one final opportunity to evaluate all aspects of the veneers before they are permanently bonded to the tooth. After you give your dentist permission to proceed, the veneers are bonded into place. Any extra cement is removed, and the veneers will be checked to be sure that they are smooth all over.

Veneers are an excellent option if you are unhappy with your smile. Your teeth can be whiter, straighter, and more esthetically pleasing in a few weeks. With proper care and hygiene, they will last a very long time.

Is it Always Correct to Save Teeth?

DO you remember how often your dentist pushed you to save a tooth? It seemed like saving teeth was always the best thing to do, and in the past it was. We developed whole specialties of dentists whose jobs it was to save teeth. Periodontists, people who specialize in gum disease, were there to help you save your teeth from the ravages of gum disease or periodontal disease. Endodontists did root canals on teeth whose nerves had died as a result of deep decay. This was good and gave many people the opportunity of chewing with teeth for a much longer period of time than they ever had before. We have lots of periodontists and lots of endodontists who do that today. I am one of them. But the emphasis on saving teeth has changed.

While it was almost "save a tooth at all costs," it isn't that way anymore. The simple reason for that is that if you try to save a weakened tooth at all costs, there are times when "all costs" may mean that you will lose the tooth, and that really costs!

Let's assume that a tooth has periodontal disease, has decay, and is fractured. To save that tooth would require a periodontist, an endodontist, and a restorative dentist. There can be up to four different procedures done on a tooth by these three individuals to save that tooth. So you would have a tooth that is weakened by gum disease and decay and that has a dead nerve. Picture a wall in your shower that has tiles coming off, water soaking through the drywall, a plumbing leak, and rotted 2x4s. How much repair can you do to an old pipe, to old studs, to old drywall, and to old tile? There is a time when you just have to replace the wall, right? A tooth is no different. Sometimes a tooth is so weakened that there is only one thing you can do, and that is to replace the tooth.

The reason we don't save teeth as much as we did in the past is simply because we have a better solution in many cases, and that is dental implants. After all, a dental implant is a replacement for a rotted root. The root of a tooth that has been ravaged by periodontal disease, or has been ravaged by decay, or is brittle because of a dead nerve can almost always be replaced with a root that is made out of titanium, a biocompatible metal, that doesn't decay, that won't break down, and for all practical purposes is much stronger than a rotted root no matter how well restored.

Here's a story that illustrates the question:

> Laura lost a tooth because of decay. It fractured, and had I tried to save it, I would have had to change her gum line as a result of removing the supporting bone to expose more tooth structure. She had a broad smile and showed lots of her gum tissue. Had I changed her gum line, I would have permanently disfigured a beautiful woman. She didn't want to have the adjacent teeth ground down for a permanent bridge (a wise choice). Why? The average bridge lasts about 7 years before further damage to the supporting teeth occurs. According to a study reviewing the literature, 11% of teeth involved in fixed bridgework ultimately need root canals. And once a root canal is done through a bridge, the chance of that bridge failing increases dramatically. Her best choice—a dental implant. In fact, Laura was able to have her dental implant and temporary crown placed on the same day as she had her tooth extracted. I extracted the tooth and placed the dental implant. Laura then immediately saw her dentist for the temporary crown. She was whole again with a pretty tooth in three hours.
>
> All dentists are trained to save teeth. It's almost automatic to refer a patient to an endodontist (root canal specialist) when the decay goes so deep that the nerve is exposed. Sometimes though, it's better to look at this badly diseased tooth before considering the root canal and ask:
>
> **Is this tooth really worth saving? Would a dental implant be more predictable?**

So while it is customary to think about saving a tooth, you should ask your dentist the question, how much will it cost to save the tooth and how reliable will all of those treatments be? Will a dental implant be more predictable and ultimately less costly? Will a dental implant more likely preserve the bone than all of the procedures that are necessary to save the tooth?

If we ask those questions, we may not only be in a better position to make a decision, we may also have a restoration that is as long-lasting as possible.

The Cracked Tooth

ONE day, I was in my chiropractor's office. He has that great candy at the front desk, the kind that you are supposed to let dissolve in your mouth. I can't do that. Maybe you can't either. I have to chew it. Well, I did chew it and all of a sudden, I was chewing on more than the hard candy. I was chewing on part of my tooth

That led me to this column because for fifteen years prior to that incident, that tooth would bother me every once in a while when I bit down the wrong way. It had a small crack, but I lived with it.

So let's go back to the beginning. How can a tooth crack? It can crack for any one of a number of reasons. The tooth itself can be inherently weak and can split right down the middle, well below the gum line, even if it's never had a filling. There is nothing that can be done to save a tooth that is split deeply below the gum line. It should be removed and is usually best replaced with a dental implant.

A tooth can crack because it is weakened by tooth decay. Tooth decay undermines the structural integrity of the tooth. Often, that crack will occur above the gum line. We drill out the decay and put in a filling to restore the tooth. But essentially now the tooth is divided by the filling. Remember when you lived up north and when the snow melted in the spring, there would be potholes in the road? Road maintenance would fill those potholes with asphalt. But what happened to those pothole repairs? They'd often have to be redone the next year because the walls of the pothole expanded and cracked, leaving a bigger pothole. The same thing happens with a tooth with a filling. The walls of the filling, meaning the remaining tooth structure, expand and contract, and cracks develop. Sometimes, it hurts to bite down on the tooth because there are "micro cracks" that are so small and so deep that we dentists can't even see them.

I am often asked the question, "How can my tooth still hurt when I had a root canal done on the tooth?" After all, the nerve of the tooth has been removed. How can it hurt? The answer is that the periodontal ligament around the outside of the tooth also has nerve fibers. So while the inside of the tooth may be nerve-free because of the root canal, the outside of the tooth under the gum line still has its ligament holding the tooth to the bone. The fracture touches that ligament. So if you notice pain when you bite down, the fracture is likely touching the ligament and "stretches" it under biting pressure.

If you feel some slight, intermittent discomfort only when you bite down and can live with it, it may be best to do just that. But if you feel severe pain when you bite down and it is interfering with your eating lifestyle, something needs to be done. Dentists will often place a temporary crown to see if the pain in the tooth is relieved before asking you to invest in major dental work on the tooth. If the pain goes away, then the investment in the permanent crown may be worth it. But if pain on biting pressure remains after placing a temporary crown, it may be better to extract the tooth now than to invest in more procedures to "save the tooth."

A year and a half later, I visited by chiropractor again. He had the same candy. I chewed it instead of dissolving it, and I fractured another tooth. You'd think I'd learn.

Before You Do the Root Canal…

Here's the scenario:

YOU'RE in the dentist's office. You have a cavity. You're numb. The dentist starts the procedure of drilling away the decay. He or she finds that the decay hits the nerve. The next statement might be, "I'm sorry, but the decay has gone too deep. You need a root canal."

Here's another scenario:

Your dentist takes an x-ray. It might be a routine check, or you may have a toothache. He/She finds an abscess or a trapped infection that is located in the bone. It's plainly visible on the x-ray. He/She says, "You need a root canal."

On the inside of every tooth root, there is a hollow tube or canal. Inside that tube are small blood vessels that nourish the tooth and nerves that allow us to feel cold sensation. The blood vessels and nerves are sensitive to bacteria, so if a bacteria-filled cavity comes close to the nerve, you may feel some pain. Those bacteria may also infect the blood vessels and nerves, causing them to die. That's where the term "dead tooth" comes from. The bacteria do not just stay in the tooth. They can travel up though the canal and infect the bone that surrounds the tooth. A root canal procedure removes the nerve from the tooth and cleans out the infection from within the tooth. It is very successful at controlling such infections.

So it would seem logical that if there is an infection in the tooth or if decay has reached the nerve, a root canal should be done. But hold on. Not so fast.

Root canal procedures are very successful, but the long-term success of the entire tooth has very much to do with the strength of the remaining tooth structure. In other words, if you have a tooth that has been badly broken down by decay or has substantial filling material in it, then that tooth is a weakened tooth. The more tooth structure that has been lost, the more decay that is in the tooth, and the more filling material that is in the tooth, the weaker the tooth is. The weaker the tooth, the more prone it is to fracture.

There is one other factor involved. The blood vessels in the canal provide moisture to the tooth root. A tooth without those blood vessels becomes brittle. What happens when you lose moisture in your skin? That's right. It cracks. A tooth treated with a root canal is exactly the same. While it does save the tooth, the tooth is more likely to crack.

Therefore, the questions that you as an informed consumer should ask are, "How restorable is the tooth? Is there sound, healthy tooth structure above the gum line? If I save the tooth with a root canal, what are the chances that the tooth will remain sound?"

If the tooth is not easily restorable, a dental implant is often the most reliable alternative.

Root Canal after a Crown Is Only a Temporary Repair

IF you need a root canal after a crown has been done, it is often only a temporary fix. This is explained in a letter to a question that I received on my website.

The question was this:

Dear Dr. Sheldon,

I have a long-standing bridge. I recently was diagnosed with an abscess on one of the teeth supporting the bridge and had a root canal done. Now there is decay on the tooth next to the one with the root canal, and I'm told to remove that tooth from the bridge. What is the risk of such a procedure?

Mary

Dear Mary,

There are some considerations that I want to take a bit of time to develop. Thanks for sharing your history with me.

The fact that you had a root canal done through the bridge and that a tooth is going to be separated from the bridge may preclude your having a temporary fixed bridge

I'm going to take the liberty to draw some pictures here, which I hope will clarify what could be going on. I hope that the pictures are clear enough to communicate the point.

I'm going to graphically draw an eight-unit bridge as I perceive you have described it.

For orientation, we'll designate the parts of the tooth and the parts of the bridge. First is the tooth. "Crown preparation" means the part of the tooth that remains after the tooth is ground down for the bridge. I'll develop the point using a single tooth and then extrapolate that to the bridge.

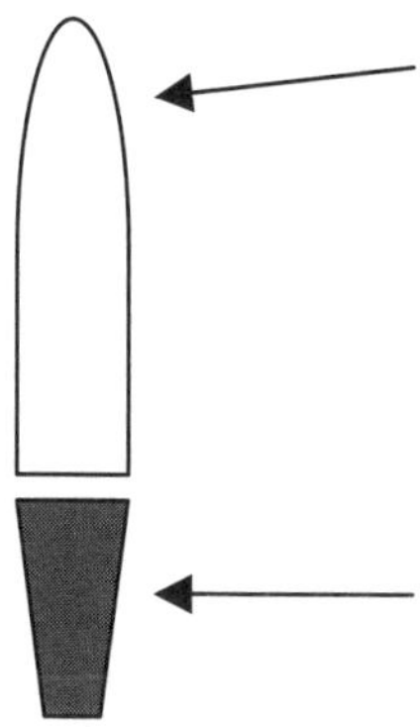

Let's now add the crown to the crown preparation.

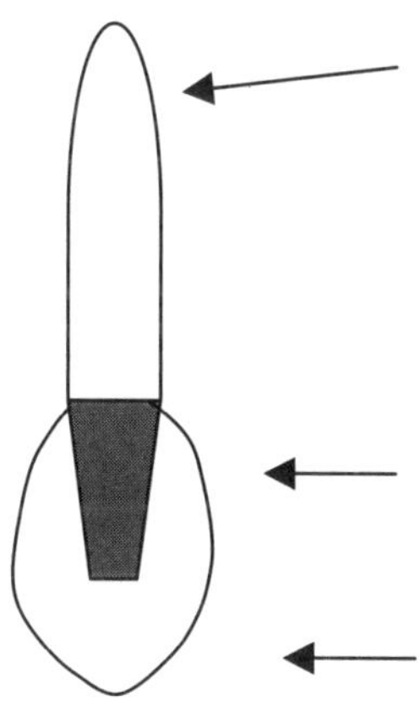

So the crown is placed on top of the crown preparation and cemented in place.

Let's assume that this is the canine tooth that needed the root canal that was done through the bridge. The dentist has to make a hole through the bridge and consequently make a hole in the crown preparation to get to the root canal.

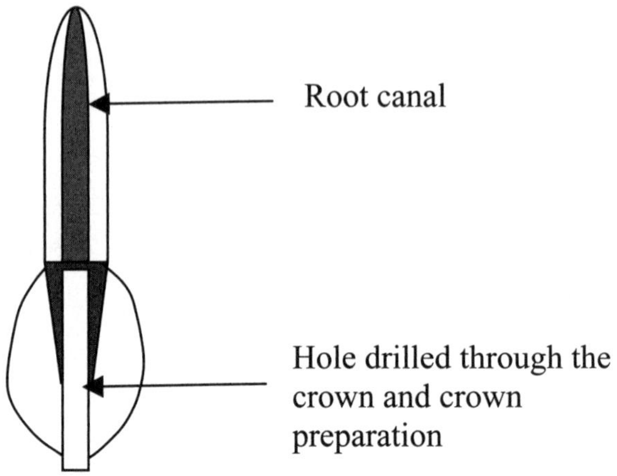

So now the tooth is weakened by the hole that was made in the center of the tooth to gain access to the root canal.

Now let's extrapolate to the entire bridge. The original bridge looks something like this, correct?

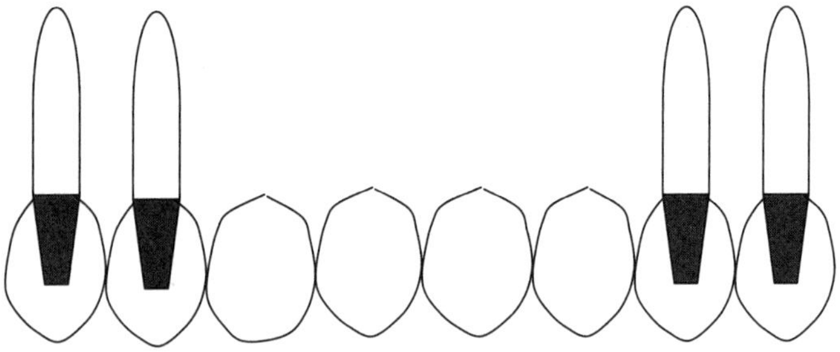

Now let's add the hole for the root canal. It is not unusual for weakened tooth structure to fracture over a period of time with continued use.

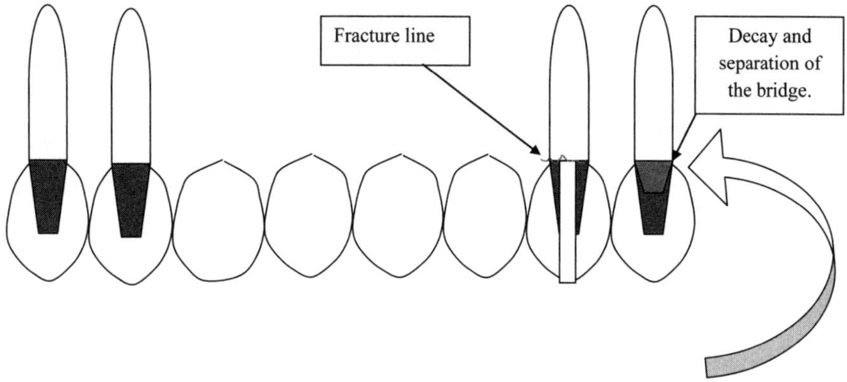

The next step is for the bridge to work itself loose from the adjacent tooth, often resulting in tooth decay.

The next step is for the bridge to work itself entire loose from that side, ultimately loosening the teeth or loosening the bridge on the opposite side. That could result in loss of those teeth.

I hope that this helps you. With the failure that is occurring, my recommendation is that you have the entire bridge attended to now rather than risk further failure.

Sinusitis Won't Clear Up? It Could Be Your Tooth.

OVER 13% of Americans suffer from some form of chronic sinusitis. This is one of the most common medical complaints, costing 6 billion dollars and 13 million doctor visits a year. While many sinus infections are self-limiting (will go away by themselves) or are easily treated with antibiotics, there is a group of patients for whom sinus infections is a way of life. And one of the previously hidden causes for such sinus infections is now coming to light, offering new hope to those who thought there was no answer.

Studies done by the Ferguson group of otolaryngologists at the University of Pittsburgh Medical Center initially looked at 5 patients whose treatment of sinusitis through endoscopic sinus surgery had failed. The elusive cause—a dental infection. What was interesting is that three of the five patients had already been screened for dental infections and were told that they had no dental pathology. The difference was a CT scan, because the CT scan can detect pathology that might otherwise be missed with conventional dental tests and x-rays. These patients were then re-treated with extraction of the offending tooth or teeth along with sinus surgery. All five patients' sinus symptoms resolved.

The group then looked at a sample of 186 patients who had previously had CT scans taken for sinusitis adjacent to the upper jaw. The findings were clear. Many of the infections were of dental origin. What was even more significant was that the more fluid there was in the sinus and the more serious the sinus disease, the more likely it was to be due to an infected tooth. How significant? A total of 86% of the acute severe sinus cases showed a dental origin.

The message is a telling one. First, the CT scan is much more diagnostic for a tooth-sinus relationship than was previously thought, and we need to look at that possibility more carefully. Second, we cannot always rely on conventional dental testing to diagnose a possible dental source of a sinus infection.

From a personal perspective, I have seen much more evidence of sinus pathology related to teeth since the advent of the dental cone-beam CT scan (CBCT).

If you have a sinus infection that hasn't resolved, these findings could be significant for you. The action that I would take would be the following: Talk to your ENT (ear, nose, and throat) surgeon. If your CT scan was taken recently, ask that a new review of the scan be done to look for a possible dental source for your infection. If that is still unclear, get a dental CT scan taken and have it reviewed both by the dentist as well as a dental radiologist. If a dental infection is the source of the problem, a cooperative dental/medical approach may help you.

DENTAL IMPLANTS

Ten Facts You Need to Know if You Are Wearing Dentures, Partials, or Are Missing a Tooth or Teeth

Fact #1: Natural teeth functioning against a denture or partial denture often cause the bone to be lost under the denture.

SARAH was a woman in her 60's who was referred to us by her general dentist for a dental implant consultation. Sarah was bright and energetic. She was hopeful that something could be done. She had been missing all of her upper teeth for so long and had a few lower front teeth supporting a removable partial denture. I looked at her mouth and was shocked to see that all of the bone in the front of her upper arch was missing. That meant that the only thing between her lower gums and her nose was...her nose. Now that might sound funny, but I don't mean it to be. Sarah was in dire trouble. As a result of her chewing with her lower front teeth against her upper denture, the ridge under the upper denture had completely worn away.

Now not every case is as bad as Sarah's, but the problem of pressure resorption is one that we see very often. Some teeth have been extracted. There are a few opposing natural teeth. The pressure from the natural teeth causes the opposing ridge to lose its bone under the denture or partial denture. People perceive it as loosening upper dentures, pain in the gum under the nose, or sore spots under the lips. Sometimes, they don't feel it at all, and the bone loss continues to worsen.

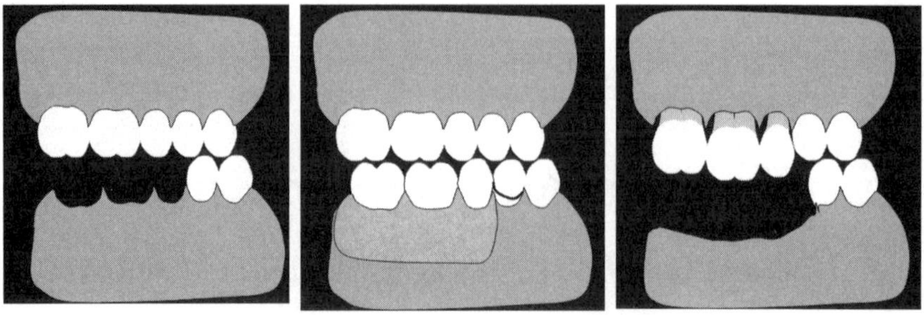

Fact #2: Loss of bone occurs in almost every case where there are missing teeth and may worsen over time under dentures.

James got his dentures years ago. They were better than the rotting teeth that couldn't be fixed. He got along with his dentures just fine, until they loosened. He tried relines and even had his dentures remade from time to time. Each time, they became more and more difficult to fit, and it was more and more difficult for him to chew, particularly on his lower denture. Why? Because the bone was resorbing in his case as it had in Sarah's. You see, the bone that we have in the jaws is there to support the teeth. Once the teeth are gone, the bone gradually leaves, too.

Fact #3: It isn't enough to just consider preserving a tooth. We must also consider preserving the bone.

Laura lost a tooth because of decay. It fractured and if we had tried to save it, we would have had to change her gum line. She had a broad smile and showed lots of her gum tissue. If I had changed her gum line, I would have permanently disfigured a beautiful woman. She didn't want to have the adjacent teeth ground down for a permanent bridge (a wise choice). Why? The average bridge lasts about 7 years before damage to the supporting teeth occurs. Her best choice—a dental implant. In fact, Laura was able to have her dental implant and temporary crown placed on the same day as she had her tooth extracted. I extracted the tooth and placed the dental implant. She then immediately saw her dentist for the temporary crown. She was whole again in three hours—no pain medication and a pretty tooth.

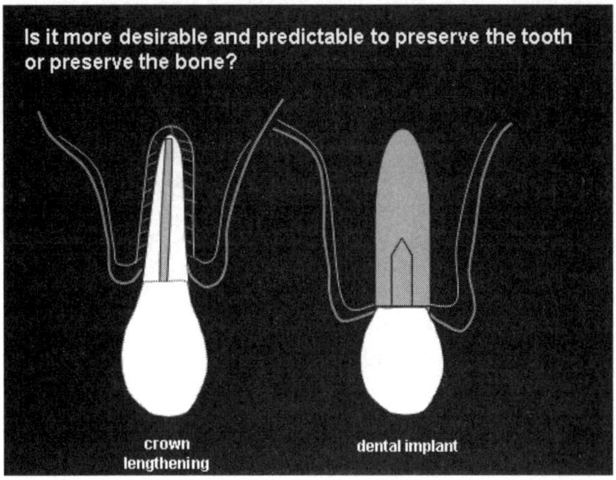

Fact #4: A dental implant, if placed at the right time, preserves bone tissue and helps to stop bone and gum shrinkage.

Jim had a single front tooth extracted after several attempts to save it failed. He decided to replace the missing tooth with a fixed bridge. Over the next few months the gum shrunk in the area where the tooth was extracted so that the tooth in the final fixed bridge overlapped the gum tissue. This created an unnatural look.

How could it have been treated instead? The tooth could have been extracted and an immediate implant placed. With an implant in place, the bone is not as likely to resorb. If the bone remains, the gum tissue remains as do the natural contours. The key is to make the appropriate diagnosis first and as quickly as possible, and then do everything we can to preserve your gum and bone as we proceed with a gentle extraction and a dental implant.

Fact #5: Teeth continue to erupt if they don't have anything to stop them.

John had his back lower teeth extracted. It was too expensive to save them. After all, they didn't show. What happened as a result? The upper teeth that were chewing against the lower teeth that were extracted started to drop down, changing the appearance of his bite. The teeth then dropped down so far that there was no room to replace his lower teeth when he finally decided that he needed to replace them.

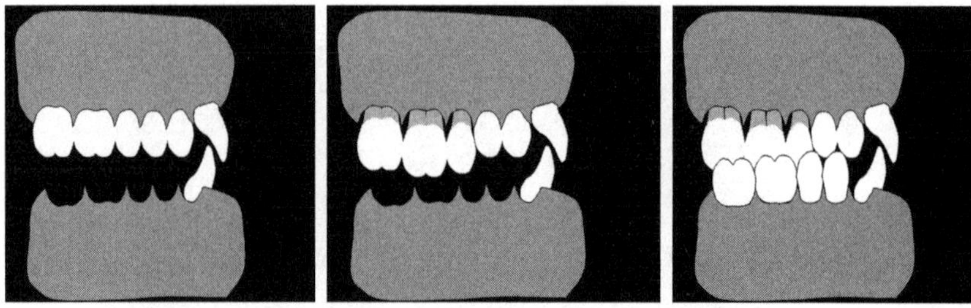

Upper teeth erupt into the empty space

Leaving no room for the opposing teeth

Dental implants placed at the appropriate time hold the bite in the correct relationship, saving damage to the teeth as well as expense.

Fact #6: The cost of an implant to replace one tooth and a cemented bridge to replace one tooth are similar, and…dental implants are more predictable than fixed bridges.

The decision on tooth replacement is a personal one. Nearly every tooth in the mouth can be replaced with a dental implant. A dental implant allows the tooth to be replaced without the need to touch the adjacent tooth. The dental implant supports the tooth itself rather than relying on the adjacent natural teeth for support. Some problem will occur in most natural tooth fixed bridges within seven years. Dental implants are more than 95% successful in most areas of the mouth over a ten-year period of time. The cost of a single dental implant and crown is similar to the cost of a bridge.

Fact #7: Nearly everyone has enough bone for a dental implant. If some bone is missing, it can easily be replaced in almost every case.

"I don't have enough bone for a dental implant," Marie exclaimed. "My dentist who saw me years ago said that he looked at the x-ray, and there's not enough bone." We hear this frequently. The facts are these. One cannot just look at an x-ray to determine whether there is enough bone. And frankly, even if you could get all the information from an x-ray, almost every area in the mouth with missing bone can have its bone replaced. Some of the bone grafting procedures that we do can be done at the same time as the implant is placed. That's how predictable they are. With the advent of the dental CT scan that allows us to see your bone in three dimensions, we often can find bone that we couldn't see previously on conventional dental x-rays. If you want dental implants, you can have them done in every area of every mouth. The only question is how much treatment is necessary to get there? Most of the dental implants that we place require no separate bone replacement procedure. It's a simple surgery.

Fact #8: The dental implant surgical procedure is painless, and people often need no pain medication afterwards.

"That didn't hurt at all. I didn't have to take any pain medication," Julie exclaimed at her post-treatment visit. There is the impression out there that dental implants are painful. It's just not true. Dental implants as a whole are the most comfortable surgery that we perform. While not everyone does this in the absence of any pain medication, most take a mild tablet for comfort the night of the implant placement, and that's it. No more pain. The reason is simple. The dental implant is usually done with a minimal need for surgery. The incision is tiny. Sometimes, particularly for a one-tooth implant, the patient does not even require stitches.

Fact #9 Allergies to the materials in modern dental implants are very rare.

"Can you be allergic to a dental implant?" was the question. The implants used in the mouth are made out of titanium or titanium alloy. This is the same material commonly used for hip and knee replacement. Loss of a titanium implant due to allergy is rare.

When an implant fails, it usually fails due to infection at the time of the surgery. If so, it is handled by removing the implant, allowing the area to heal, and redoing the implant. This is a very infrequent complication and occurs very early in implant therapy. The worst that would ordinarily occur would be a delay in the completion of the dental implant.

All-ceramic implants may be an effective alternative for those with metal sensitivities. However, they are "one piece" implants. Therefore, they have prosthetic limitations and may not be able to be appropriately adjusted in many situations.

Fact #10: The dental implant is strong, doesn't fracture or decay, and is predictable.

"Can you save the tooth?" the patient asked. That's an important question. The question that we should also ask is how much work will it take to save the tooth? How much damage will result to the bone in saving the tooth? What's the risk of the tooth fracturing later on? How predictable will that approach be? The answer is this: If it takes only one procedure to save a tooth, that's pretty predictable. The more procedures that it takes to save a tooth, however, the less predictable it becomes. Each procedure has its rate of failure. As procedures increase, so do the opportunities for failure. A dental implant is strong, doesn't decay, and fractures only in the most stressful situations, such as strong tooth grinding or trauma. For those who grind their teeth excessively, damage to an implant-supported restoration can be mitigated by your wearing a protective appliance called a nightguard.

Bonus Fact #11: Missing back teeth will cause the front teeth to shift and/or wear.

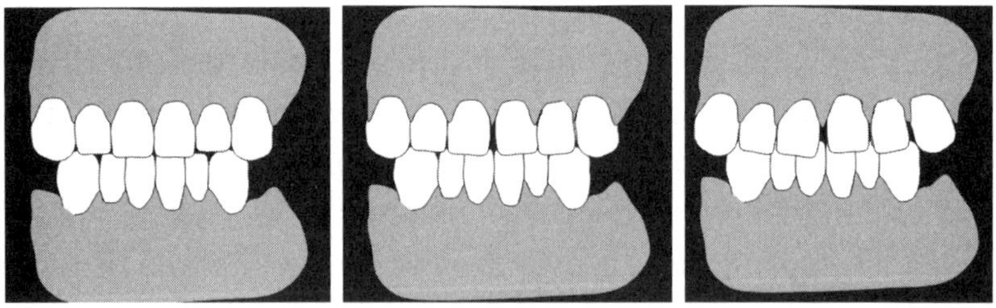

It's Not the Denture

IT happened in our office again just last week. And seemingly, it happens almost every week. Here's the line: "I've just had a denture made, and it doesn't fit right." I check it, and it fits as well as it's going to fit. What's the problem? Often, it's not the denture. It's you.

Now this is not an excuse for a denture that doesn't fit right. That sometimes happens too, and with minor corrections, that can be remedied. This is for the person who says, I've never had a denture fit as well as the first one.

Now why would that be? Denture materials, if anything, have improved over the years. The impression materials that we use likewise have improved. (And wait. They're getting even better, with electronic digital impressions slowly making their way into everyday dentistry. No more goop. No more waiting for plaster models to be poured and trimmed. It's already here and will be in common use in the next few years.)

The denture impression procedure is critical, and this is a skill that most dentists master in dental school. So if it's not the materials, and it's not the dentist, what could be the problem?

The minute the teeth are extracted, the bone that held the teeth shrinks away. For some, it's a gradual shrinkage. For others, it's more dramatic. For almost all, the shrinkage continues over time, simply due to the pressure of the denture on the ridge. Every time you bite down, every time you clench your teeth, you are placing pressure on the ridge. And that pressure results in shrinkage of that ridge. We call it "ridge resorption." Did your dentist tell you to take your dentures out at night? It was to help prevent shrinkage of the ridge, because we often clench our teeth at night.

The ridge shrinks, and of course the denture doesn't. So what else happens over time? Do you notice that the lower third of your face is shorter? That your chin is closer to your nose? That's because of ridge resorption. Do you notice that your lower jaw juts out when it didn't before? Same thing—ridge resorption. How about your nose sticking out farther than it used to because your upper lip puckers in? Ridge resorption again.

Here are some methods that help limit ridge resorption.

1. Save your natural teeth, if you can save them predictably.
2. If you wear dentures, take them out as much as possible and certainly at night.
3. Get dental implants, preferably as closely as possible after you lose your teeth.

Resorption starts on the first day that you lose your teeth. Denture wearers are often the people least likely to see the dentist on a regular basis. But the need for dental care never stops. Your dentist can check for resorption, reline or remake your dentures, and adjust your bite to minimize the damage that may otherwise occur. Don't let the loss of your teeth stop your dental visits. Just as you need your physician to monitor your health, you need your dentist to monitor your oral health.

Case Story

When one is missing his/her lower teeth, it literally creates a "dental cripple." The lower ridge is very thin. The tongue moves, the lips move, and the denture unfortunately moves as well.

Harry went to several dentists and several surgeons to look at all the options available. After several weeks of looking and comparing options, he decided to have the work done in our office. Here's what Harry has to say about his procedure:

> *"I had my teeth out when I was 19 and had dentures until I was 66. I should have had implants many years ago. These new dentures, secured by the lower implants, are excellent and allow a much more secure chewing and talking atmosphere. I researched the implant world for several years and finally*

> *decided to trust my very low-profile ridge to Lee Sheldon. I have been happy with the results and trust that the future now looks much brighter than the past, regarding personal appearance and comfort." – Harry*

He wrote that in 1999. At this writing, it is now 12 years later and his implants are still functioning beautifully.

The Three Dangers of Tooth Loss and Poor Fitting Dentures that You Must Know About!

Danger #1: Wearing dentures causes accelerated bone loss. This results in the loss of support of your facial muscles, causing you to look older much more quickly.

YOU'VE seen denture wearers. They are constantly moving their mouths to position the denture, particularly the lower denture, in the right position. And as pressure is transferred from the denture to the bone, the bone resorbs. Not only does the denture not fit, but the bone resorption results in loss of support of the face. The lips become thinner. The chin moves closer to the nose. The final result is a nose and chin that stick out while the mouth and cheeks sink in, with wrinkled skin and deep folds in the corners of the mouth which remain continually inflamed. Moreover, the combination of wrinkled corners of the mouth along with saliva often results in a fungal infection.

Danger #2: Poorly fitting partial dentures increase your risk of tooth loss and gum disease.

Partial dentures depend on the underlying gums for support. Often there are clasps placed to allow the partial to be partially retained by the natural teeth. Pressure on the partial denture causes the underlying bone and gum support to be gradually lost. When that happens, there is more stress on the clasps, resulting in more stress on those teeth. The teeth often loosen as a result. The partial denture also "sinks" as the bone support is lost. It then rubs against the gums, causing gum and bone loss around the natural teeth.

Danger #3: Dentures may reduce your life span.

You know what you're eating now. You know what foods you avoid. Often the foods that you avoid are the very foods that you need. When was the last time that you comfortably ate a fresh vegetable, bursting with nutrition? And 8-10 servings of fresh fruits and vegetables a day are the exact prescription for cancer and heart disease prevention. Imagine having teeth that felt close to your own, that didn't shift, and that you could actually chew with. You wouldn't shy away from those healthy foods again, because you could now chew them.

"Solid Bite" Hybrid Dentures Can Alleviate Dental Woes

YOU have a bad tooth. You go to the dentist and get a filling. Then the tooth hurts. You need a root canal and a crown.

That's OK if it happens once or twice, but what happens if you go through this sequence again and again? Are there other answers?

Yes, there is another answer—an answer that doesn't involve decay and has a better success rate than any form of tooth replacement: a dental implant. Along with the implant, you'll need a crown and a post to hold the crown onto the implant.

OK, you say, a dental implant will work, but I'm having this problem again and again and again. I can't afford a dental implant for every tooth that goes bad.

Well, there's lots of good news here. You don't have to replace every bad tooth with an implant.

Other people who have bad teeth, rather than continuing to replace them, opt out of the dental system. They wait for the ultimate to happen, and then they think that they'll have to have dentures. Why? Dentures are less expensive, they don't wear out readily, and they seem to be the only option.

What would happen if you combined the lower cost of denture materials with implants? You would have a tooth replacement system called a hybrid, a dental implant-supported denture with all the security of implants supported by bone, and a denture fastened to those implants. It wouldn't move and wouldn't cause denture sores. We call it "Solid Bite."

It would be smaller, so the roof of your mouth wouldn't be covered. You would chew almost the way you did when you had healthy, natural teeth. You wouldn't need to have your dentures removed if you had surgery. You wouldn't have to think about what you could and could not order on a menu. And, in the event that a tooth broke, it would be a simple repair.

Implant-supported hybrid dentures are nothing new. They've been around for more than 25 years. They're generally used to replace full arches of missing teeth.

Almost everyone who is missing teeth still has enough bone support for a hybrid. And with modern dental CT scans, we can often find good implant-supporting bone we couldn't see on traditional x-rays.

So, if you've been missing teeth for years, you still qualify for a hybrid. Hybrids are cost-effective, amounting to roughly half of what a full arch of implant-supported crowns would cost.

Some of our happiest patients are those who have found an answer to the continual downward spiral of dental disease. They found Solid Bite, and are smiling and chewing better than they have in years.

Here is a Success Story from one such patient, Veronica O'Brien.

> *"When I was diagnosed with diabetes six years ago, I started having a lot of problems with my mouth and periodontal disease. I came to Dr. Sheldon and the only way to treat the problem was to lose all of my teeth. So we went through a two-step process. First [was to] remove the top set, replace it with implants, and get the upper bridge put in. Then we did the bottom set eight months ago. And now my mouth is fully healed. I don't have the problems that I was having with the dry mouth, with the constant fungal infections. I can talk. I can eat. I can smile. My teeth look better. These are my teeth. The benefit of receiving the full bridge replacements versus the cost, you really can't compare, because I was having so many problems with dry mouth and trouble eating and my teeth shifting that it was becoming more of a hindrance than a help. So when I look at the cost versus the hindrances that I had, there is just no comparison. It is an investment that you are making in yourself and that's what's important.*

The staff in Dr. Sheldon's office is absolutely fantastic. They're very caring. They really take the time to get to know you as an individual, which really makes it nice. And I, you know, I can't say enough about them. They're just absolutely fantastic girls and I love every one of them.

This office is different because they take the time to know you. So when I call up and I say, 'This is Veronica O'Brien,' anyone answering the phone knows that it's me and knows that I am a patient and knows basically the treatment that I have been under so they can help me get the information or the help that I need at the moment.

Compared to three years ago, my life is so different because I can actually smile and be confident with my smile. I can eat. I can sleep. I just feel healthier all around because I think your health system starts in your mouth to begin with, and it goes down the rest of your body.

My life is different now with eating and smiling because I can actually smile. Three years ago I could not smile. I did not feel the confidence in opening up my mouth and letting people see my teeth. Now I can let people see my teeth. With eating I can actually chew something and not worry about being in pain. I wasn't able to chew before without being in pain, so that's how it has changed.

I was having a lot of trouble smiling because my teeth were moving around in my mouth. They were decaying. I was, like I said before, I was having trouble eating. Now I don't have the trouble eating. Now I can smile and be confident and be able to do things that I wasn't able to do before. I don't have the problem of being in pain all the time which was a big issue for me.

Dr. Sheldon is very professional. He is very easy to talk to. He is willing to listen to what your opinion is. He works with you to figure out which is the best course of treatment that you should have. He is very open to listening to what you'd like to achieve and he is willing to work with you. This process was always done at my own pace and how I needed it to be done." – Veronica O'Brien

Solid Bite Immediate: Using Technology to Speed the Result and Reduce Surgical Trauma

What do our patients want?

- Fast service
- Less surgery
- Fixed prosthetics

Let's be specific. We now have the technology to place implants and teeth all in the same day. Additionally, by utilizing CT scans and computer software, all the surgery can be done on the computer first, maximizing the use of your supporting bone and designing the teeth to have outstanding immediate function. This means that we don't have to make incisions to see the bone. It means that there is almost no bleeding or swelling. What else does it mean? It means that you can have your dental implant surgery in the morning and be eating at a restaurant that evening.

What do we call this? Solid Bite Immediate. What does Solid Bite Immediate provide?

- Teeth fixed in place on the same day as dental implant surgery
- Flapless surgery which means almost no post-operative discomfort and swelling

The following pages show you the details of the procedure:

1. A denture is modified for the CT scan process.
2. A CT scan is taken with the denture or a tooth mock-up in your mouth.

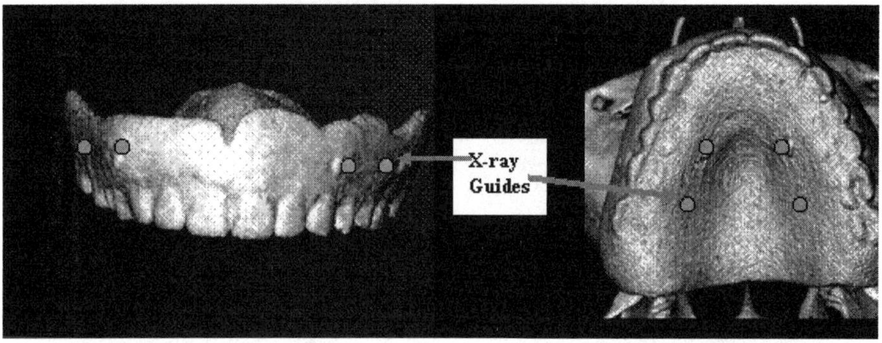

3. I can then see the CT scan of the bone and the teeth on our computer.

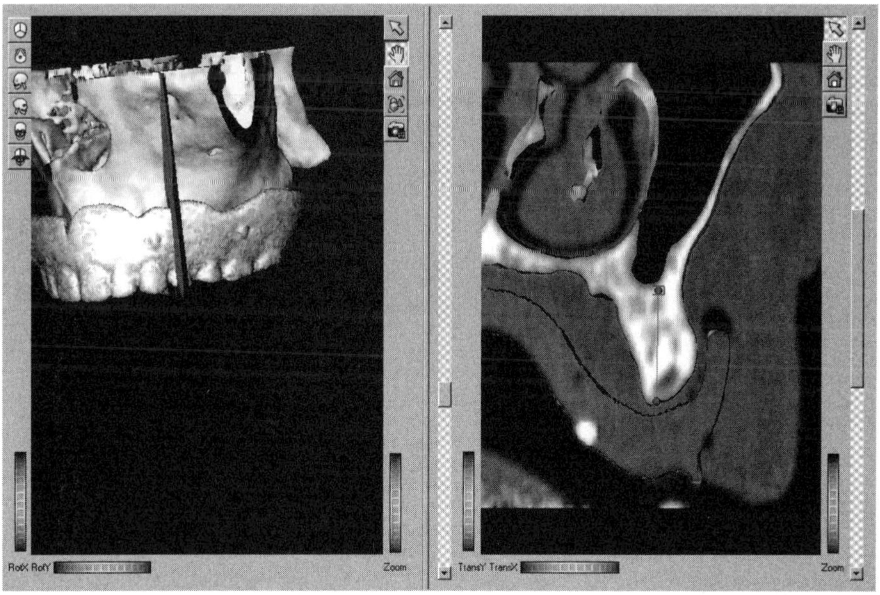

4. Using the CT scan, I design the placement of the implants, using the best available bone and angulation.

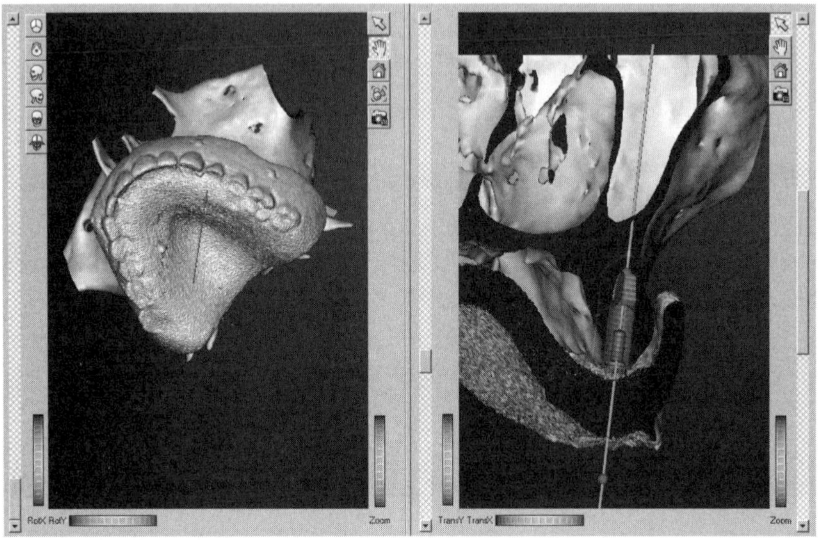

5. Design is completed. This design shows 6 implants. Three retaining pins are designed to stabilize the surgical guide during implant placement.

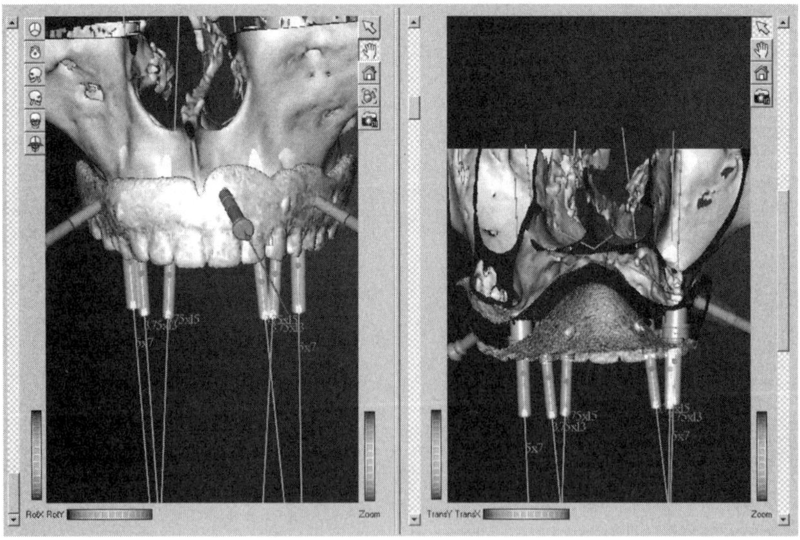

6. The plan is then sent electronically to the laboratory. The laboratory then makes a surgical guide so that the implants are placed in the exact, predefined position on the computer.

7. On the day of treatment, six implants are placed, with no incisions and in less than an hour. The dentist can then place temporary fixed teeth directly on the implants. You can be chewing that evening.
8. You chew with the temporary teeth for 2-6 months, to allow time for the implants and bone to heal. Your dentist then makes permanent teeth on the implants.

Do you have to be missing all of your teeth for immediate tooth replacement to apply to you? No. In many cases, we are able to extract your teeth, place implants, and place temporary teeth on the implants in the same day. If you have enough bone support, this can be done. It is a standard part of the examination in our office.

Here is a success story from one of our Solid Bite Immediate patients.

"These teeth are actually better than my teeth. There is a certainly psychology, I think, tied into it. I think there's times when the body intelligence maybe doesn't like a certain part of itself. It didn't like my teeth. And when Dr. Sheldon put these teeth in, oh, it was like beautiful from day one. Needless to say, you could walk right out and start eating a steak if you wanted to. The advice I would give would be this, you have to ask yourself, as the old saying goes, "Are you sick and tired of being sick and tired?" And you know if the teeth haven't bothered you, well fine, you don't have an argument. But if you have problems and you are spending a lot of money, and it's like putting a Band-Aid on a cancer, the best thing to do is come in and have the original teeth taken out, put these teeth in, and you'll be happy forever. Initially up front it may appear to be a lot of money, but in the long run you save money. And it's the happiness that goes with it.

The whole thing is so comfortable, it's unbelievable. So if somebody were to ask if there was any pain associated with it, I would have to say that there wasn't. Was there discomfort? No there wasn't.

You come in here and you feel like family. You feel like they're happy you're here. And of course that gives you a good feeling.

The quality of life, I guess, is lack of suffering. The suffering has gone away, where you always have that probably at a subconscious level. It was always back there, the gums were always sore, the gums were always bleeding, you always had periodontal problems. There was an anxiety tied in with it because you were looking ahead to the next time you had to have periodontal work, which is pure suffering. I would never go through it again. I would go ahead, step right out, have the job done, and be happy forever after, let's put it that way.

As far as Dr. Sheldon, he's probably.... he's a walking genius. There's no doubt about it. I mean he is extremely well organized, extremely knowledgeable. He's a very person's person—very, very dedicated to this. I mean, he has a natural calling for this... You couldn't feel any more confident with anybody. He has a very positive, upbeat personality." – Robert Redfern

Solid Bite Premium: The All-Zirconia Solution

THE basis of the Solid Bite approach to dental care is to create an all-implant supported solution for the upper and lower arches for patients whose dental longevity with natural teeth is limited. Natural, healthy teeth are better than any dental implant solution, but for those teeth that have been ravaged by decay, periodontal disease, and root canals, an implant solution is often more predictable than saving those teeth.

In a previous chapter, we talked about the Solid Bite hybrid. No, this isn't a hybrid car with large batteries taking over for the gas engine, but like a car, the hybrid is a combination of technologies. In this case, it is the use of three different materials to create the Solid Bite hybrid solution. Those three materials are a metal substructure for strength, pink acrylic to simulate your gum tissue, and pre-fabricated denture teeth, which beautifully simulate your natural teeth. It is a sight to behold. Solid Bite is comfortable, durable, and strong, and if there is a fracture of some of the acrylic material, it is easy to fix.

As good as the Solid Bite hybrid solution is, the three different materials can separate, particularly if you are a tooth grinder. In addition, acrylic can accumulate stain over a period of time from coffee, tea, wine, and smoking. There is a solution to those problems as well: Solid Bite Premium.

Solid Bite Premium is the culmination of years of technological research to develop an all-ceramic solution for full-arch tooth replacement. It is constructed out of a single material, Zirconia, which is both strong and durable. Through the use of computer CAD-CAM technology, a single piece of strong Zirconia is milled to create a beautiful prosthesis. Gum tissue color almost totally matches your gum tissue. Teeth are custom designed, and most importantly, there is no possibility of separation of the three materials because Solid Bite Premium is made of a single material.

Zirconia is considered the most durable material for single crowns. Take a sledge hammer to an all-Zirconia crown and the crown doesn't even chip. Imagine constructing an entire arch with that same material. Add to that customized, layered porcelain on the front teeth to create an individualized smile and you then have natural-like beauty as well as strength.

What is the risk? There is always a risk of breakage of an all-Zirconia prosthesis, and because it isn't easy to repair, that risk may be a costly risk as well. While the risk of fracture is very low, if it does break, the prosthesis needs to be remade. The good news is that the laboratory has a computer record of your prosthesis, so the cost is not the same as making the prosthesis from scratch. Because Solid Bite Premium comes with a temporary bridge, which we will give to you, the broken prosthesis can be easily removed and the temporary placed by any dentist who has some facility with implants.

You have the choice of prostheses. Once you see your choices, you'll see how close we have come to creating a beautiful and functional Solid Bite.

The Ceramic Dental Implant

THERE are times when something new comes along that may make an impact on implant dentistry. As I've done implant dentistry for nearly my entire career, I have seen things come and go. Procedures and material arrive with great promise. Some succeed, some fail, and while I'm very excited about the ceramic implant, I want to be careful to "under promise" and when I possibly can, to over deliver.

The ceramic implant is made out of a crystalline structure called zirconia. Zirconia has been used for dental prosthetic restorations, like crowns and bridges for many years. One of our concerns about ceramics has been its strength and resistance to fracture. Zirconia bridges have been quite strong, and zirconia crowns are now leading the way in resistance to fracture. In fact, the all-zirconia crown is now the restoration of choice for people who grind their teeth.

The zirconia implant that we use is the Ceraroot, which was developed by a family of dentists, the Olivas, in Granolliers, Spain, in 2004. They have taken pains to use a zirconia material that is the leader in the market for strength and safety. They have also had tests done at the University of Minnesota that demonstrate high bone compatibility, no inflammatory changes in the bone and soft tissues, and biologic attachment that is similar to that of the bone and gum tissue with a natural tooth. Over 3,000 Ceraroot implants have been placed worldwide with no evidence of fracture.

The Ceraroot implant is different from conventional dental implants. In other chapters of the book, we've described the conventional titanium implant as being a three-piece system: the implant, which is a titanium root that's placed in the bone; the abutment, which is a post that is screwed into the implant to hold a crown; and the crown itself.

The Ceraroot implant is a one-piece implant. That means that the implant and the abutment are one solid piece.

The Cararoot implant has its advantages and disadvantages.

Here are the advantages:

- It has a built-in abutment.
- It is white in color and esthetics may be improved, particularly in "thin gum cases."
- It is biologically inert.
- There are no demonstrated allergies to zirconia.

Here are the disadvantages:

- The bone has to line up perfectly with the missing tooth.
- The patient has to be careful to keep the tongue and food away from the implant while healing.

So let's go into a bit more detail regarding the ceramic implant and its advantages and disadvantages. One tremendous advantage with the titanium implant is that if there is bone loss or angulation of the bone, I can place the implant at that angle and then correct for that angle with a custom abutment. Let's say your bone is angled at 30 degrees from normal. I can place that implant at a 30-degree angle. Later on, I can place a corrective abutment so that the crown lines up perfectly. Because the zirconia implant is one piece, I can't do that. If the bone is angled, I have to correct that angle with a bone graft first so that I can place the zirconia implant without an angle. That problem is encountered more often on the upper arch than the lower. It's another reason why a pre-operative CT scan with planning software is so necessary. We can do the surgery on the computer before we do it in your mouth and know what problems we may encounter and plan appropriately.

A titanium implant is placed below the gum line so the chances of traumatizing an implant during healing are very small, but the zirconia implant sticks out of the gum tissue. Implants need to heal without trauma. I remember very well a patient came to me two weeks after placing an implant and told me that it was loose. I asked him how he knew. He said, "I kept checking it with my tongue, and sure enough it got loose."

Implants need to heal into the bone passively. New bone needs to form into the threads of the implant. The tongue is a strong muscle, and yes, it can loosen a perfectly good implant, so we really need to be careful of a zirconia implant and make sure that it's allowed to heal passively.

Other than the above, a zirconia implant is beautifully esthetic. It heals beautifully with the soft tissue, and all indications—and I say that with some reservation as there are not a lot of us placing these implants yet—are that they may be the most biologically compatible implant on the market today.

You DO Have Enough Bone for an Implant

IT happened again. A patient comes into my office and says that she was told that she doesn't have enough bone for a dental implant. There may have been a reason to say that 20 years ago...but now?

There are two major advances which make a lack of bone a thing of the past: 1) the method of x-ray diagnosis and 2) the graft materials to help you replace missing bone.

Let's first consider the x-ray. The traditional x-ray provides a view of your mouth in two dimensions. It can reveal height and width. It can't reveal thickness, the third and most important dimension. The way we see that third dimension is with a CT scan. Yes, there are dental CT scans, made specifically to determine bone availability for dental implants. An additional benefit is that dental CT scans produce only about 2% of the radiation of a medical CT scan. CT scans give us a complete surgical view of your bone before we do the surgery. I can't tell you how often I find good dental implant-supporting bone in a CT scan that I am unable to see in traditional dental x-rays.

What's even better is that we can do your dental implant surgery first on the computer, and design a template from that virtual surgery that we place in your mouth, making your actual surgical procedure easier and faster.

While improvements have been made in dental implants since the basic design was introduced in 1982, the monumental improvement that has occurred lies in the materials available to graft bone. There are dental bone powders that are used to fill extraction sites to prevent bone shrinkage. There is bone putty that we place on your existing bone to increase its thickness. There are blocks, and wafers, and sponges, all designed for the same function—to restore missing bone. There are methods to harness the growth factors from your blood to increase the speed of bone healing. There are also materials that recruit your own stem cells from surrounding tissue to produce new bone, as well as grafts that have "built-in" stem cells.

So whether your sinus is too low or your bone has diminished, or you've been told that you don't have enough bone, there are answers for you.

No bone? Get a dental CT scan. Once the diagnosis has been made, the answers are simpler and more predictable than ever before.

Biologic Modifiers Enhance Surgical Results

WERE you told that there is no solution for your gum disease? Have you been told that there just is no room for dental implants? New technologies are now available giving new hope to seniors who won't smile and can't chew.

One of the rapidly progressing advances is the area of "biologic modifiers." These are products extracted from your blood or from human or animal sources that improve your ability to heal.

The fact is that growing new gum tissue has never been easier or more predictable. Gone are the days when we tell you that you don't have enough bone for a dental implant.

So let's cover gums first. There are freeze dried tissues that we literally can take from an envelope, hydrate them, and place them in the mouth to grow new gum tissue. And what appears to enhance their healing even further are your own platelets. Your platelets have growth factors, and through the use of a centrifuge, we can concentrate these growth factors, add them to the graft tissue, and increase healing, predictability, and comfort of soft tissue grafting procedures.

For lost periodontal support, there is an enamel derivative taken from animal sources that enhances the replacement of periodontal support. That has been around for several years. A more recent product stimulates your body to introduce its own stem cells to the tooth-bone interface, enhancing bone growth even further to restore bone support for the tooth.

Bone enhancement to increase bone support for dental implants has never been better. In the back of the upper jaw, the sinus has been a barrier to placement of dental implants. The "sinus lift" procedure, which changes the position of a low sinus, has been providing new bone support for dental implants for years. These procedures have been improved through special tools that reduce the size of the bone incision. Bone modifiers improve the outcome even further. Taken from animal sources, they provide a substance called bone morphogenic protein, which acts as a magnet to draw your stem cells to the area. Your stem cells then grow the required bone and gum tissue. If your bone is too narrow, there are laboratory- fabricated membranes that form the scaffolding for the new bone, so that narrow bone can become wider bone, usually within a period of four to six months. That allows for dental implants to be placed. Often, the dental implant and the bone graft can be placed simultaneously, cutting down the time it takes before you get your new implant-supported tooth.

And the dental CT scan makes the procedure even easier as we can now "find bone" that we are unable to identify on conventional dental x-rays. Imagine being able to do "virtual surgery" on a computer before ever having the procedure done in your mouth. We can do that. Imagine doing a bone graft and an implant at the same time, reducing the number of surgical procedures and the time from missing tooth to final restoration. We can do that. Imagine breaking a tooth in the morning and replacing it with a dental implant that same day. We've been doing that for years.

If you've said to yourself, "I wish I could eat normally again, "the solutions are easier and more predictable than ever.

Advancing Dental Surgical Technologies Help All of Us

I'VE been back from a trip to Spain for less than twenty-four hours. The trip wasn't a pleasure trip, although my wife and I had a good time. The trip was a professional trip for additional training in the latest technologies in bone regeneration and dental implants, and did I get back pumped!

Some of the latest scientific advances in dental surgical technology are originating in Spain. A technology called PRGF®, Plasma Rich in Growth Factors, has been developed over the past fifteen years by a thorough and scientific dentist, Dr. Eduardo Anitua. Dr. Anitua not only is the director of a comprehensive dental facility, he also employs a staff of biologists, pharmacologists, and other scientists to advance the science of bone and soft tissue regeneration. His staff of three hundred in the small city of Vitoria has advanced the research of tissue regeneration utilizing the growth factors from a patient's own platelets to do such things as regenerate bone and soft tissue of the mouth. But it goes farther than that as he is contributing to the medical literature using the same technology to heal large diabetic ulcers, repair injured tendons, and provide facial rejuvenation, all utilizing the patient's own growth factors.

And of course that's what all of us in the health professions are there for: to improve our patients' lives. It is special people like the Dr. Anituas of this world that make our lives better. He not only creates the solutions, he advances the technology and employs a group of scientists to verify the validity of his work and help in its expansion. He then publishes the research in top medical journals, where the data is reviewed and verified. He does this with no government grants, no pharmaceutical money.

On to Barcelona to visit a family of dentists, the Olivas, who over ten years ago saw a need and developed a ceramic dental implant. There is an increasing demand for metal-free restorations, including metal-free dental implants. The Olivas recognized that growing demand, and they set out to do research into the ceramic zirconia. They also followed the scientific method, testing not only clinically but also in the laboratory, to confirm that such an implant could work, and what they have produced is an implant that more closely mimics the body's own bioelectric properties. Zirconia has been verified as a biocompatible material.

This is clinical research. They apply the technology by placing the implant, and then publish their results. They employ outside researchers to verify the validity of the product that they have developed. Their latest research was done at the University of Minnesota, showing excellent bone-to-implant contact. I even assisted on a case. My assistants would have been proud to see that their boss knows something about their side of the chair. Then I reviewed with one of the doctors, case after case after case. They document everything, showing me what they did in unique situations to create a successful result.

It is the innovators of this world who expand our horizons and improve our lives. They don't see barriers; they see opportunities. They don't see failure; they see stepping stones to success. They improve the science and share their excitement as well as their technologies with the world, and that excitement is contagious.

Look Carefully at New Technology Before You Start Treatment

THOSE of us who choose the leading edge in health care do so because of the word *leading*, but the word *edge* may be more important to you. An edge is sharp and, unless used precisely, can hurt. An edge has nothing beyond it to return to. And finally, an edge has no base, and in this case, no base of experience.

So let's look beyond the glitz of the newness. Maybe the tried and true is a better fit for you. But whether it's the shiny new technology or the tried and true, there are more basic factors to look at.

1. What is the level of competence of the person providing the service?
   Have you spoken to others who have had the service with that particular individual? How carefully have you looked into that practitioner before you are enticed by the technology?

2. What is the experience base of that person in that technology?
   Some of us are more experienced at some procedures than others. It's perfectly okay to ask the practitioner whom you are considering how much experience he or she has with that procedure and what the results are.

3. What happens if things go wrong?
   The new technology may result in fantastic successes and applications that have never been available in the past, but there are also new challenges with that technology that could

be discovered during your treatment. What happens if the leading edge becomes too edgy for you? Are you prepared for those challenges?

4. Diagnosis is much more important than treatment technology. We are all enamored with the treatment itself, the new gadget, the micro-micro instrument, but the secret to successful treatment is not necessarily the gadget; it is the diagnostic process. The gadget may be great, but if the thought process doesn't cut it, neither will the gadget.

5. A treatment plan is often more important than the treatment itself. We can talk in dentistry about the crown, the bridge, the root canal, or the implant, but how does that treatment plan fit into your total mouth picture? What will happen to the adjacent teeth? What additional expectations and expenses does the doctor predict for the rest of the mouth?

6. What is the condition of the body (and mind) of the person who is receiving the service, and how willing is the person to improve that condition?
   Your success is not only treatment dependent, it's also patient dependent. We can repair the ravages of disease, but we can't change the cause of the damage. That's your job. We can advise you, but the bottom line is what you are going to change to help ensure treatment success.

7. Are your expectations greater than what the practitioner can deliver?
   People sometimes expect more than we can deliver. Both the patient and the doctor should have clear communication before treatment starts so that both are happy at the end. If the doctor finds that he can't deliver what the patient wants, then there may be a new technology just over the horizon that will work. But then you will be on the *leading edge* of technology again, and you know how that goes.

Does Your Lower Denture Wobble? Fixing it is "A Snap."

ONE of the true enjoyments many of us have in life as we age is eating. We may have more time to cook, or we just look forward to going out to eat. Some of us enjoy eating more than others. Why? Many have a lower denture that wobbles, and no matter what they do, that lower denture just doesn't feel right.

It's a problem for denture wearers, and the question usually goes like this: Why does my upper denture feel secure, while my lower denture doesn't?

The answer is in your anatomy. You have a palate on the upper arch, a large area where your denture rests. And because of that, the upper denture fits like a suction cup. The lower doesn't work that way, because your tongue is in the way. The lower denture just doesn't stand a chance with a tongue whose muscles move when we talk, when we swallow, and when we eat.

In previous chapters, I've talked about dental implants to replace an entire arch (upper or lower) of teeth with teeth that are fixed in place. These are great, but may not be affordable for some. There is, however, a solution that may do just enough to make you comfortable and start enjoying your food again. It's the two-implant "snap."

A two-implant snap works this way. Two implants are placed into the front part of your lower jaw, spaced about an inch apart. Included in those implants are receptacles that hold a snap—the same kind of snap that holds a jacket together, the same kind of snap that fastens an infant's clothes. The other part of the snap is then attached to the inside of the denture. So instead of the denture floating up and down, it now snaps into place. Two snaps are the minimum. A good candidate for the two-implant snap has some remaining lower ridge and enough room in the existing denture to hold the snap. If you want additional snaps in the back for even more stability, they can be placed at the same time or added later on.

The surgery for the two-implant snap is minimal, sometimes not even requiring an incision. And it won't break the bank, costing $5-7000, depending on the quality of the lower ridge and the usability of the existing denture.

Our bodies thrive when we eat the correct foods. If you are changing your food choices because your dentures just don't do the job, think "snap."

Case Story

What are the benefits of dental implants? Dental implants are not just posts. They have the potential for changing one's life.

Read a Success Story from a patient of ours, Leigh Anne.

> *"I have never been the type to gamble or play the stock market, but if I did, I would have invested in the product 'Fixodent.' Literally, I went through a couple of tubes a month. Even then I 'couldn't leave home without it!' After each meal I would have to re-glue. I lived this way for the past 11 or 12 years. I didn't think that I would or could enjoy food again. I just thought that this was the 'norm' for all denture wearers. It got to the point to where I would even have to re-glue after eating a peanut butter and jelly sandwich.*
>
> *So I went to see my dentist to see what I could do about my predicament. He told me about a new way to wear dentures and never needing to wear adhesive again. I thought, 'Yeah right,' but I listened anyway. He set me up an appointment with Dr. Sheldon and explained the whole process called 'dental implants.' Little did I know this would be my ticket back to the 'Garden of Eatin(g)' after all these years. As the a proud owner of a set of implants, I then took a bite out of the best and most*

> *expensive apple I have ever eaten and boy was it worth the wait and any amount of money. As a matter of fact, it was worth every pretty penny I ever earned.*
>
> *I am biting into every kind of food I enjoyed when I had all of my own teeth.*
>
> *Dental implants are truly the next best thing to having your own teeth. As a matter of fact, I am eating better and healthier food now that I am able to enjoy "Mother Nature's best!"*

Here is another Success Story:

Bonnie is 61 years old. She had all of her teeth extracted at the age of 21, and still was using her 40-year-old dentures. Over the years, Bonnie had lost much of her denture-supporting bone. As a result, the lower part of her face was shrunken, giving her an appearance that was far older than her years. She couldn't chew. She had had her dentures relined three times with no improvement. On the day of the examination, she sneezed and her dentures flew across the room.

She had two implants placed with snaps connecting the implants to her new lower denture. She also had a new conventional upper denture made.

> *"When I first came to Dr. Sheldon, I could not eat very many foods. My mouth dipped way in... I couldn't wear lipstick because I had no lips.*
>
> *Now I can eat anything I like, even steak. It is so great! I'm not ashamed to go out to eat, [or go to] parties or weddings.*
>
> *For a long time, I wouldn't go anywhere. But now I am very proud of the way I look. Thanks to Dr. Sheldon and his staff."*

Little did I know that when I first started doing dental implants 25 years ago that it would be any more than tooth replacement. The fact is that these success stories are common. People find that their lives change, simply as a result of being able to chew their food again. They are able to select the foods that they want rather than the foods they are required to eat because of the limitations of their teeth. This is actually one of the most gratifying experiences of my practice life, to be able to change a person's life for the better.

The One-Piece, Same-Day Dental Implant

THE lower denture is uncomfortable for nearly every person who wears one. Why is the lower denture a problem much more often than the upper? The upper is made as a large suction cup that covers the entire palate. It takes advantage of a large surface area to seal it to the surrounding tissue.

But the lower denture doesn't have nearly that kind of support. The only support that it gets is from a pencil-thin ridge. Often that ridge is sharp, producing sore spots. That ridge gradually deteriorates, reducing the denture support even more. When the tongue moves, the denture moves. When you pronounce some words, the lips dislodge the denture. And if you laugh or sneeze? You'll have your hand over your mouth immediately not because of good manners, but because you're afraid that the denture will fly out of your mouth.

There are dental implant supports available for an existing lower denture, the simplest being the one-piece implant. The one-piece implant has two basic components, a screw-like portion that goes into the bone and a snap-like portion that emerges from the gum. The big bonus in the one-piece implant is that the entire procedure is done in one day. The implant is placed, and the existing denture is relined chairside with a silicone material that engages the "snap" in the implant. You literally walk in with a floating denture and walk out with teeth that are snapped in place.

Here are the requirements for a one-piece implant–supported denture:

1. a denture that has good occlusion (bite) with the opposing arch
2. a denture that does not rock when firm pressure is placed on it
3. a dental CT scan so that the dentist can see the amount and shape of the bone (This allows the dentist to plan the length and diameter of the implants as well as diagnose the best positions for the implants to be parallel.)

This can be done on the upper arch as well. We usually use four to five implants on the lower and five to seven implants on the upper, depending on the amount of supporting bone that is present.

The procedure goes like this:

The dentist makes a small incision into the gum area and removes any rough areas of bone that could cause irritation. A small hole is made into the bone. The implant is screwed into place. The remaining implants are then placed in a similar fashion. Small stitches are then placed. These stitches melt away in a few days.

The inside of the denture is hollowed out to create room for the silicone reline material. The reline material is placed into the denture and then in the patient's mouth, allowing it to set over the "snap" portions of the implants. The denture is then removed, excess silicone is trimmed away, and the denture is seated back in the mouth. The entire process takes less than two hours. It is not unusual for the periodontist or oral surgeon to do the implant surgery and for your general dentist to do the reline.

After healing is complete, you remove the denture and clean it once a day, just as before.

The one-piece implant allows you to stop thinking about your teeth, allows you to eat foods that you've been avoiding, and gives you the confidence to talk, smile, and laugh, knowing that your denture will not come loose. It has helped thousands.

Dental Implants: Questions We Are Frequently Asked

Q: What are dental implants?

A: Dental implants are replacements for the roots of the teeth. They act as anchors to support a tooth or many teeth. Dental implants are constructed from titanium or titanium alloy, the same materials used in hip and knee replacements. Implants are also available that are all-ceramic.

Q: What are the benefits of dental implants?

A: Here is a list of just a few of the benefits:

1. **They prevent bone loss.** By preventing bone resorption, which would normally occur with the loss of teeth, the facial structures remain intact. This is especially important when all of the teeth are missing, because the lower one-third of the face collapses if implants are not placed to preserve the bone.
2. **Overall quality of life is enhanced with replacement teeth that look, feel, and function more like natural teeth.** You will look younger and more attractive, and this allows you to be even more confident and enjoy smiling, laughing, and talking with others.
3. **You may live longer because you'll get to eat better and prevent malnutrition or stomach problems!** Fresh vegetables and fruits are back on the menu! You can now eat the foods you like. Also, since your chewing is improved, your digestion will be even better as well!
4. **They increase the amount of enjoyment you get out of eating.**
5. **They create more confidence in social situations.** Most of our

patients love their new implants because of their improved appearance, function, and comfort.

6. **They allow you to relax and not have to worry about your dentures moving around, popping out, or gagging you.** You'll never worry about your dentures flying out when you laugh, sneeze, cough, or when you eat. Implants are so securely attached that the fear of dentures falling out will be eliminated!
7. **Your mouth will be restored as closely as possible to its natural state.** By replacing the entire tooth, as well as the tooth root, it is possible to replicate the function of natural teeth with a strong, stable foundation that allows comfortable biting and chewing. Also, nothing in the mouth looks or feels false or artificial!
8. **You will be able to taste foods more fully.** Wearing an upper denture can prevent someone from really tasting food, as the roof of the mouth is covered. With implant-supported replacement teeth, since it is not necessary to cover the roof of the mouth, you can enjoy the taste of foods.
9. **They eliminate the need for denture adhesives.** Since implant-supported teeth are securely attached to the implants, there is no need for messy denture adhesives.
10. **Your other teeth will not be altered to replace the missing teeth.** Since replacing missing teeth with implant-supported crowns and bridges does not involve the adjacent natural teeth, they are not compromised or damaged. For example, when you wear a partial denture, you have clasps that hook onto adjacent teeth, which put pressure on them and can cause them to wear, break, loosen and/or come out. Additionally, bridges require grinding down the adjacent teeth so that the bridge can be cemented on them. This tooth structure can never be replaced and the long-term health of these teeth is compromised.

Q: Am I a candidate for dental implant treatment?

A: Almost anyone who is missing one or more teeth and is in general good health is a candidate for dental implant treatment. There are a few medical conditions that can undermine the success of implant treatment, such as uncontrolled diabetes. However, there are few conditions that would keep someone from having implant treatment altogether.

Quality and quantity of available bone for implant placement is more often a factor in qualifying for dental implants than medical conditions. However, even people who have lost a significant amount of bone can qualify for dental implant treatment with additional procedures to add bone or create new bone. Advances in this type of treatment have made it possible for thousands of patients who would not previously have been considered candidates for successful implant procedures.

In addition, the new dental CT scans allow us to "find" bone that we cannot see on conventional dental x-rays.

Q: How painful is getting dental implants?

A: There is no pain during the procedure. In addition to traditional local anesthetics, another option that many choose is conscious sedation, using intravenous medications. In our office, we are fortunate to have two assistants who are IV certified, as well as a medical anesthesiologist available to us. Our office has been doing IV conscious sedation throughout my career. You will be comfortable for the entire procedure.

Q: What else do you do to ensure my comfort during treatment?

A: Our office provides headphones with music, warm blankets, and intravenous sedation. Equally importantly, we have an experienced staff that is dedicated to making sure that things go right for you.

Q: What do you do to ensure my safety?

A: Our entire staff is CPR certified, and Dr. Sheldon is certified in

Advanced Cardiac Life Support as well. We have an automated electronic defibrillator (AED) as well as emergency oxygen and medications. Because we do IV sedation on a regular basis, our staff is well-trained to handle any problem that may occur.

Q: How long will it take to complete the treatment?

A: You will notice a difference almost immediately. However, the entire process can take between 2 and 9 months to complete. In cases requiring bone grafting, it may take a little longer. This depends on the type and quantity of implants you need, along with the quality of bone in which the implants are placed. If you fracture a front tooth, we can often place an implant and a temporary on the implant on the very same day.

If you are missing many teeth, you can often have teeth extracted, implants placed, and temporary teeth secured to the implants on the same day.

Q: Is it possible to have my tooth extracted, my implant placed, and have a tooth placed on the implant all in the same day?

A: Yes. Immediate implant placement is becoming more popular as the technology improves. We can determine your candidacy for immediate implant placement during your consultation visit.

Case Story

What happens when you break a front tooth? The first thing is often panic. Rhonda had that problem. She had lots of options in regard to replacing that tooth. One would be to place a temporary partial denture, which is something that is removable and fits over the roof of the mouth. It pops in and out, just like an orthodontic retainer would, except that it has a tooth on it rather than a wire. Rhonda chose the immediate implant option.

Essentially, what happened was that she walked in, we took out the tooth, put in an implant, and put a temporary tooth on the implant all in the same day. Here's what she writes:

"When I broke my tooth, I was given several options, but

chose to have Dr. Sheldon do a dental implant. At 10:30 am Dr. Sheldon pulled the broken tooth out, extracted some bone from my back jaw, and performed the dental implant in 45 minutes! I then went to my dentist and he put on a temporary crown at 3:00 pm! I was hesitant about doing it all in one day, but I went back to work teaching 19 kindergarteners the next day!! Everything went so smoothly and I would recommend it to anyone! Dr. Sheldon and his staff are friendly, efficient, and professional!" – Rhonda C

Q: Will I need to have one implant placed for each tooth that is missing?

A: No. In fact, it is possible to replace all of the lower teeth with an over denture that is supported by only 2-4 implants. On the other hand, it might sometimes work to your advantage to replace your back teeth with an implant for each tooth to provide additional strength. For a full Solid Bite case, most patients require 5 implants on the lower arch and 6 implants on the upper arch. The treatment chosen depends upon your desires as well as the amount of available supporting bone.

Q: How do I know if I'm too old for implants?

A: Great question. Your overall health and your desire to improve your quality of life are much more important things to consider than your age. The ages of our dental implant patients have ranged from 16 to 98 (yes, 98). As you age, there are fewer and fewer things to enjoy in life. Chewing your food can be one of the last pleasures you have. You probably have seen aged people struggling with their dentures, or losing their dentures, and then have nothing left to chew with. You've seen the embarrassment that accompanies this as children and grandchildren visit them, seeing Grandma or Grandpa without teeth for the first time. And unfortunately, by that time, nothing can be done. Dental implants placed now can help assure you that you will be able to chew, that you will have teeth for the rest of your life.

Q: How long do implants last?

A: Most research has shown that the vast majority of implants last for over 20 years. Our goal is to have them last a lifetime.

Q: What is the cost of implant treatment?

A: Many people call us and ask, "How much is one implant going to cost?" While I wish the answer were that simple, the only way to determine actual cost is by having you come in for a consultation and examination to find out if you have bone loss and exactly how many implants you will need. The actual cost of implant treatment is based on a number of factors, such as the number of teeth being replaced, the type of treatment option recommended, and whether additional procedures are necessary to achieve the proper esthetic and functional results. You can simply donate $50 to our Charitable Giving Campaign, described in another section of this book, and you will receive an examination and x-rays (excluding CT scans and complex treatment planning) at no charge. We'll be able to give you an estimate during your first visit with us.

Q: Why should I see a periodontist for my dental implant treatment?

A: Most periodontists do surgical treatment nearly every day. The periodontist is also intimately involved in determining which teeth can be predictably saved and which cannot. The periodontist, therefore, is also a treatment planning specialist. Your general dentist and periodontist meet to determine a treatment plan that is best for you. In other words, you get an instant second opinion. Together, both dentists will create a treatment plan that is best for you. Very often, particularly when a patient has some teeth, there is the need for gum treatment to help save those teeth. There are times when we can save a tooth rather than replace it with a dental implant. By seeing a periodontist, your gum treatment can be done at the same time as the dental implant treatment, saving you time and money.

If you don't have a general dentist, we will find one who is perfect for your situation.

Q: Do I have to change general dentists if my implants are being placed by a periodontist?

A: Definitely not. In our particular practice, we have worked with well over 100 doctors in dental implant therapy. Such dental teams are common and result in great care. If you don't have a dentist to place teeth on the implants, the periodontist can select one for you that will fit your needs. The periodontist knows the qualifications of the local general dentists and can select the right one for you.

Q: What if I don't have a dentist?

A: We know the dentists in our area and can select a dentist for you that will provide an excellent result.

Q: What advances are there that can make my treatment even more predictable?

A: There are several to include:

1. **Digital x-rays**—The digital x-ray provides immediate feedback during the surgical procedure so that the surgeon knows the correct angulation and the precise length of the dental implant. There are times when several x-rays are taken to assure proper placement of the implant. Conventional X-rays might take as long as 6 minutes to process. With a digital x-ray, the picture shows up on the computer screen instantaneously, providing instant results as well as shortened surgical time.
2. **Plasma Rich in Growth Factors (PRGF)**—This is one of the newest advances that is being used in plastic and orthopedic surgery as well as in dental surgery. Your own platelets, the part of the blood responsible for forming a blood clot, have numerous growth factors that can accelerate healing of the treatment site. Just a little of your blood, taken from your arm at the time of surgery, is processed in our computerized

laboratory centrifuge to separate out these platelets. The platelets, when added to bone grafts or soft tissue grafts, speed healing of the site, increasing your comfort and minimizing the need for pain medications.

3. **Bone Morphogenic Proteins (BMP)**—Synthesized BMP's placed in combination with bone grafts stimulate the recruitment of stem cells from other parts of your body to move to the grafted site, stimulating bone production in grafted sites.
4. **Dental Endoscope**—This tiny camera, placed below the gum line, allows us to see many areas that are ordinarily not accessible to the naked eye. Particularly useful when treating natural teeth, the endoscope adds to the predictability of the procedure. It literally helps us "look around corners."
5. **Surgical Microscope**—The surgical microscope helps in visualizing incision lines and surgical repair, particularly in areas of cosmetic concern, so that you can have smaller stitches and better closure of the site.
6. **Cone-beam CT-Scan (CBCT)**—The CBCT provides you with a three dimensional view of your jawbone. By seeing this third dimension, we can much more easily locate good implant supporting bone as well to more precisely plan your entire case. We literally can do your surgery on the computer first, saving you time, discomfort, and, sometimes, money. Radiation safely is also important. The CBCT utilizes only 2% of the radiation that a routine medical CT scan provides.
7. **Osstell stability meter**—The Osstell provides us with an objective reading of the stability of the implant in bone. Such information can tell us when the implant is ready for a tooth to be placed upon it. Often, people can have implants restored even faster because of this unique instrument.
8. **Experience**—In regard to our particular practice, *I placed my first dental implant in 1986 and have been training and educating others in dental implants ever since. Over 100 dentists have referred their patients to us for dental implants.*

Q: Does insurance cover dental implant treatment?

A: Insurance coverage depends on your individual policy. Unfortunately, most companies exclude implants as a covered benefit.

Case Story

What do you do when you have no bone? The sinus is very prominent for many people in the bicuspid and molar areas in the upper arch, and there are times where the only method is to change the position of the sinus and to place bone underneath the sinus so that dental implants can be placed. It can be done quite comfortably, and it's quite a predictable procedure. Carol had just that problem. She needed back teeth. She had periodontal disease and it just couldn't be treated any more. It came time to not only extract teeth, but to create new bone support for her new implant-supported teeth

"I had made an appointment [with Dr. Sheldon] to get a second opinion regarding gum surgery my dentist at that time wanted to do on my lower teeth. I had just recovered from having my upper mouth done.... After the exam Dr. Sheldon assured me that I did not need the surgery on the lower gums, but confirmed my upper teeth were in trouble. I had lost a lot of bone and was about to lose more teeth. It made me sick to think of all of the money I had spent on crowns, bridges, and miscellaneous painful procedures and nothing had been said about the extreme bone loss until now. I knew at that point that I needed to change my doctor. Dr. Sheldon and my new dentist (Dr. M.) came up with a plan to correct the problem.... I needed a double sinus lift, bone transplant, and tooth implants, six to be exact. (I wish I had known Dr. Sheldon earlier.) I chose to proceed ahead with the double sinus lift and bone transplant.... I can honestly say I had no pain afterwards. I did have swelling.... By the following Wednesday, the swelling was gone and on Sunday morning I was greeting at church and no one could believe I had that surgery the week before. The implants came later again without

a problem and no pain. Thanks to Dr. M., I was never without teeth. The temporary bridge I wore for almost two years looked and felt great and I could eat anything I normally ate before. My mouth has never looked or felt better!"– Carol S.

Yes, there are many times when we can do immediate tooth replacement. Very often teeth can be extracted and implants can be placed on the very same day. There are occasions when more aggressive work needs to be done. That doesn't mean you have to be without teeth. You can have good-looking and comfortable teeth for a temporary phase while the foundation work is being done. The key lies in dental treatment planning, and it's important that you, your dentist, and your surgeon have a good discussion and that all of your questions are answered before you proceed with such therapy.

When Should You Stop Seeking Dental Care?

YOU think your teeth and gums are separate from the rest of your body? Yes, insurance companies "think" that way, don't they? The fact is that every part of our body is connected. If you are a senior reading this chapter, remember the song, "The knee-bone's connected to the thigh bone...the thigh bone's connected to the hip bone...?" Nothing could be truer.

So let's look at the most recent study that demonstrates the oral-systemic connection. It was a simple study. Take 100 patients hospitalized with respiratory disease. Compare them to another 100 patients of the same age, sex, and race who are healthy. And then look at their periodontal health. What do you think I'm going to write next? Yes, the patients with respiratory disease had significantly poorer periodontal health. That means more gum inflammation, deeper periodontal pockets and bone loss around the teeth. Low-income patients had a disease rate of 4.4 times that of higher income patients. And smokers had significantly more bone loss than non-smokers.

The low-income relationship is not surprising as people with low income are much more likely to eat poorly with high levels of refined carbohydrates. That leads to increased chronic inflammation in the body and more degenerative disease, including periodontal disease. And that says tons about where our concentration in the health care arena should be. And I know that you, if you are a smoker, don't need another attack. Just consider it another reason to consider stopping.

Today, I saw a patient on emergency who had not seen a dentist in 25 years. Over the years, she had made sure that her husband and children were taken care of. She's in her seventies and has a potentially life-threatening tooth abscess approaching her eye. She knew she had problems in her mouth since 1994, when she broke a tooth. So she was in pain, swollen, and needed an incision and drainage procedure to drain the large amount of pus from her cheek and gum. She'll need a lot more help to get straightened out.

The key to this study and to this current patient is to not let your teeth go. Teeth can last a lifetime. And teeth ignored not only can cause life-threatening infections, but they can also negatively impact heart disease, diabetes, Alzheimer's Disease, and now respiratory infections. In pregnancy, periodontal disease can cause low birth-weight babies. And what would you bet that other diseases not yet studied are also impacted by poor dental health?

I was once asked a question by Joe Steckler, an advocate for seniors, on his T.V. show, "Aging with Dignity." The question was, "When should you stop dental care?" The answer then and the answer today is, "When you give up on life."

Overseas Dental Treatment? Beware!

I JUST saw this headline in an airline magazine: "World-Class Dental Services at 50–70% Savings over U.S. Prices!" A lot of other verbiage, mostly misleading, continues. Then is the kicker: "With all the money you'll save, you can vacation in style in Costa Rica."

Here's the story, one of many stories: A long-time patient of mine had the idea that he would save lots of money on dental work—much of which, by the way, he didn't absolutely need—by going to Costa Rica. Not only that, but he had also decided to become part-owner of the Costa Rican dental clinic. He had the work done. My hygienist then saw the patient, saw the dental work, and described it in a one-word term that summed it all up: *substandard*.

I then saw the patient. I look at the work, which consists of crowns on nearly every tooth. Visually it looked all right, except around the gum line, which was redder than I had remembered. Then I checked it with dental instruments to see how the crowns fit, and on crown after crown, I was able to get my examination instrument between the crown and the tooth. In other words, the crown didn't fit the tooth. Then I examined the other crowns. None of the crowns fit. Then I checked the bite. The front teeth met when he closed down, but the back teeth didn't

He was working for the Costa Rican dental clinic, so he was interested in my opinion. I said, "Let's take a set of x-rays." So we did. I had an advantage. My x-rays were digital and projected on a 37-inch video screen, so anyone could look at the x-ray and see what I saw. I showed him each crown, and rather than the crown fitting like a finely designed, custom-made restoration, they looked like a cowbell on a stick. It was obvious. It would be plain as day to you as much as it was to me. The patient, better termed "the willing victim," defended the work by saying that he "rushed the dentist." I then asked him, "Are you selling this?"

He said that he wasn't selling it yet, that he was going to be a test case before he started selling it to others. He then went on to defend himself and the clinic, telling me how cheap it was and how "this is for people who work at [a convenience store] and can't afford dentistry." He then told me proudly how much he paid for it, a bargain price.

So, here's what he received for his bargain price: crowns that didn't fit, causing gum inflammation as well as a predisposition to decay, a bite that predisposed him to jaw problems, and a greater chance of premature tooth loss.

As patients, you are at a disadvantage. You can't tell your dental condition, nor can you evaluate the treatment. Good dental work requires time and good understanding of bite relationships and their corresponding jaw relationships. It requires the understanding of how to prepare a tooth, the conditions of the nerves of the teeth, and the biology of gum disease and dental decay. It requires understanding of cosmetics and specific instructions and communication with the dental laboratory. If implants are to be considered, good dentistry requires knowledge of the shape and density of the bone as well as the relationship of the position of the bone with the position of the teeth. And with all that, things can still go wrong. They can go wrong because biology and mechanics are not always perfect. The best dentists I know immediately recognize when things are wrong and make them right. That takes training; that takes practice; that takes time; that takes *integrity*.

Where will this patient go now? He said that he'll go back to Costa Rica to have the work "done right." But if a dentist is willing to do substandard dentistry, do you really think that he is capable of doing it right? And when the patient has a problem, where is he then going to go?

To quote a popular maxim in dental circles, "Beware of bargains in parachutes, brain surgery, and dental treatment."

TMJ AND HEADACHES

But I Don't Grind My Teeth

SO a patient sits there in my chair. He's a nice guy, says that he doesn't have a problem. His teeth are just naturally short. "Really?" I said. The height of a front tooth is supposed to be greater than its width. His teeth are badly worn and are wider than they are tall. Some are even a bit loose, but he doesn't notice that.

Another patient comes in because she's broken a front tooth. She is obviously upset. No one wants to walk around with a broken front tooth. How embarrassing. And she had spent so much time and money on that tooth. Now it's broken and needs to be replaced with a dental implant.

A third patient comes into my office. She gets headaches all the time. I ask her what she means by "all the time." She says that she wakes up with headaches and that they are along the side of her head and sometimes behind her eyes. She's been told that she has migraines or maybe it's her sinus.

And then there is that fourth patient. Boy, is life miserable for him. The chewing surfaces of his teeth are sensitive. He didn't have sensitivity as a child or in early adulthood, but as he's aged, his teeth have become more and more sensitive.

So what do these four patients have in common? They all suffer from the problem of bruxism, the continual grinding of their teeth. It's not unusual. Many of us "brux," whether we think we do or not. One problem is our perception of bruxism. We think that someone would hear a loud grinding noise when we brux. That might happen in babies and small children, but when adults brux, they often grind their teeth for a few seconds, then stop, and the sound that's made is negligible. Others tell me that they snore and therefore they couldn't be bruxing, but the fact is that snorers are often bruxers, too.

When you brux, your jaw muscles go into overdrive. The nerves that control those muscles continue to fire. If you were lifting weights for fifteen minutes of every hour for eight hours a night, would your biceps be sore? The same holds true for your jaw muscles. Sore jaw muscles are innervated by the same nerve that causes headaches, so if your jaw muscles are working too hard, you may get a headache. If you wake up with headaches, what do you think has caused them? What were you doing all night? That's right: lifting weights with your jaw muscles.

How can you determine of you are a bruxer? Look in the mirror. Are the surfaces of your teeth flat? Can you see grooves on the chewing edges of your front or back teeth? Are you continually chipping teeth? Have you fractured teeth without any known cause? If so, you are a bruxer.

Fortunately, this is an easy problem to treat for most. Treatment starts with a plastic guard that is placed between the teeth. Your dentist can make it so that the forces from the bite are evenly distributed. Studies show that such an appliance reduces both the strength and the frequency of muscle contraction. Different appliances are made for different situations. To answer the question, "Can I just buy one at the drug store?" the answer is that a generic appliance cannot be adjusted and cannot direct your bite so that you minimize muscle contraction.

If you think you have a bruxism problem, talk to your dentist. Write down all your symptoms. Compare your teeth by looking at pictures of yourself from years ago. Getting bruxism treated appropriately can reduce not only headaches, but future dental expenses.

You Can Diagnose a Bad Bite. Take the LOAD TEST.

OUR periodontal practice has always seen the worst of the worst dental cases. That's not unusual. The reason that one is referred to a specialist is because he or she has needs that go beyond those that can be served by a general dentist. Sometimes, people realize that themselves and see a specialist on their own.

One of the most common complaints of my patients is that their smiles don't look the same as they used to. The front teeth are jagged. When they smile, more of their gums show, or just the opposite; when they smile, their upper teeth can no longer be seen. Another common complaint is that their front teeth have shifted. Some find that their front teeth are loose, while others find that their front teeth have fractured, even after root canals and crowns have been done. If you're still reading this chapter, I'll bet that you fall into one of these categories.

What do all of these complaints have in common? What links each of these complaints? They decided to extract some back teeth early in life and never had them replaced, or they had them replaced with a removable partial denture.

Yes, I know they are only back teeth, but back teeth provide the foundation to prevent your mouth from overclosing. If you are missing back teeth, the upper front teeth hit much harder. The lower teeth push against the backs of the upper front teeth. Those angular forces result in either severe tooth wear or loosening of the front teeth.

Another problem that may occur is that some teeth may not touch their opposing teeth when you are fully biting. So those teeth that do meet absorb more force than they were designed to.

Here are two tests that you can do right now, while reading this chapter. I call it the LOAD TEST.

LOAD TEST #1

1. Place your index finger along the front surfaces of your upper front teeth. That's it. Just put your finger under your lip and let it rest on the front surfaces of your teeth.
2. Now tap your teeth together.

Do your front teeth move a little when you do that? If so, please read on.

LOAD TEST #2

This test is a little harder.

1. Get a cellophane wrapper from any box that you have in your pantry or in your kitchen.
2. With a scissors, cut the cellophane into a strip that is about ¼ to ½ inch wide and four inches long.
3. Take that strip of cellophane and rest one end of it on one back tooth, and continue to hold the other end of the cellophane between your thumb and index finger.
4. Now close your teeth together.

   5. .... While your teeth are closed together, try to pull the cellophane out of your mouth.

   If your back teeth are touching, you'll feel a tug as your back teeth are preventing the cellophane from being removed. However, if the cellophane comes out easily, those two upper and lower teeth are not touching.
6. Try that for each of your teeth.

You'll now be able to determine for yourself which opposing teeth are touching and which are not.

If all of your teeth are touching, congratulations! If some of your back teeth are not touching, what does that mean? It means that every time your teeth are coming together, only some of them are doing the work. They are taking more LOAD than they were designed to. The fewer the teeth that are doing the work, the more LOAD each of those teeth is taking. And that means that those teeth are taking on more LOAD than they were designed to take.

It is common in our practice to see that some or many of the back teeth do not touch. And when that happens, the additional stress placed on the front teeth causes them to either shift, fracture, or become loose.

If you've had a partial denture made to replace your back teeth, it is often made of acrylic teeth, which wear over time. Think of what would occur if you wore a leather shoe on one foot and a flip-flop sandal on the other. Which would wear faster? The flip-flop is your partial denture. So while you may wear your partial denture all the time, it may be doing nothing to remove the LOAD from your front teeth. Also, a partial denture is very often supported only by the gum tissue under the partial. The gum tissue has some give to it, so when you bite down, the partial sinks a little, placing more LOAD on your front teeth.

What is the difference between a partial denture and the natural tooth it replaced? The natural tooth has a root that is attached to bone. Bone is relatively rigid and therefore, the bone supports the LOAD of your muscles when you close down. The best that a partial denture can do is to transfer that LOAD to the natural teeth that are holding the partial in place. Those teeth are not only doing more work than they were designed to, they are also being twisted and worn by the clasps that are holding the partial in place. If you've been wearing a partial for a long time, you know what I mean. If you don't know what I mean, go to a mirror and pull back your lip. Take a look!

We as dentists cannot always save every tooth. It would be great if we could, but sometimes the damage is just too extensive. In the event that a tooth is lost, it should be replaced with something that is fixed in place. The more back teeth that are lost, the more important this rule is.

Generally speaking, the most predictable way of replacing teeth is with dental implants. A dental implant is a titanium root that is attached to the bone. It can absorb LOAD stresses that are similar to those that a natural tooth can absorb. It does not decay, it very seldom fractures, and it has almost a 30-year track record of predictability. A dental implant is the most predictable way of replacing missing teeth.

So yes, it is important to control dental decay. Gum disease should be recognized early and treated appropriately. You now have a third thing to look at—the LOAD TEST.

Click in your jaw? Headaches may not be far behind.

DOES your jaw click when you open and close your mouth? This condition can worsen and cause headaches, ringing in the ears, inability to open and close the mouth.... You get the picture.

This condition used to be called TMJ (temporomandibular joint). Now it is called TMD (temporomandibular dysfunction). It really doesn't make any difference what it is called. The fact is that clicks in the jaw are not normal. Picture this. We have cartilage in every one of our joints. In the case of your jaw bone, the cartilage is between the jaw and the skull. It is there to lubricate and to allow you to open and close your mouth smoothly.

But the cartilage can become misshapen. The ligaments that hold the cartilage in place can be stretched. The surface of the cartilage and the jaw bone can roughen. All of these lead to a deteriorating condition that results in a joint click. The problem can worsen, producing jaw pain and headaches, and may be an important factor in migraines. If we clench or grind our teeth, which most of us do from time to time, that puts additional stress on the delicate cartilage, making the problem even worse.

Most of my patients tell me that they don't grind their teeth, and you may be saying the same thing right now. New research shows that when we grind our teeth, we don't grind them very loudly. The old concept of being able to hear somebody in the next room grinding their teeth is actually one that is much more the exception than the rule. Most of us grind our teeth very softly and very lightly and the grinding episodes may last five seconds or less, so nobody would hear you. But if your front or back teeth are flat, if the edges of your front teeth are three colors; white on the outside, yellow in the middle, and white on the inside, you have worn the enamel of your teeth away and could be doing damage to your joints in the process.

The treatment is rather simple, and the first stage of treatment very often involves wearing a plastic appliance which fits between the teeth. By wearing this plastic appliance, you can't close your mouth all the way. And when you can't close your mouth all the way, your joint cartilage doesn't compress either. This allows the cartilage more room and more freedom to heal, particularly at night when you clench and grind your teeth and compress that cartilage unknowingly.

The benefits of appliance therapy can be tremendous. Besides reducing tooth wear and the tendency to crack teeth, an oral appliance can help diminish headaches and jaw muscle aches.

Case Story

Marie arrived at our office with earaches and soreness in her neck. She had chronic facial pain and earaches. She also had periodontal disease.

It's interesting that after periodontal treatment alone, the soreness in her neck and ear went away. She had also experienced problems with her jaw joints and associated musculature.

> *"It was hard to believe that a little appliance that Dr. Sheldon made for me could make such a difference. At first I didn't really think that it would help much for my chronic pain, but I went from waking every night, not being able to lift my head from the pillow (the headache was <u>so</u> bad) to one headache, and a mild one, since the appliance has been first inserted. I have not experienced headaches for months.*
>
> *I had facial tingling in my cheek and pain and ringing behind my ears. I also experienced tingling and numbness down the arm and pain in the neck and shoulder. The pain in the shoulder has decreased tremendously and I am <u>so</u> happy with my results. I am very grateful to Dr. Sheldon and his friendly and competent staff."– Marie M.*

Suffering Migraines? Maybe it's your bite.

IF you've suffered from migraines, you know how debilitating the problem can be. Let's talk about the possible source of the problem as well as a possible solution.

Migraines come from an enlargement of the blood vessels in the head. Those blood vessels are commonly behind the eyes and in the areas in and around the temples. When the blood vessels engorge, they place pressure on a large cranial nerve called the trigeminal nerve, which supplies pain fibers in the areas behind the eyes as well as to the side of the head. The pressure on the nerve then results in pain. One common treatment for migraines is the drug sumatriptan, which reduces the size of the blood vessel, thus dissipating the pain.

The trigeminal nerve actually has two functions. As a sensory nerve, it produces pain. However, it also is a motor nerve, controlling functions of the temporalis muscle as well as other major muscles that move the lower jaw. Want to feel your temporalis muscle? Put the palm of your hand on the side of your head between your eye and your ear. Now clench your teeth. You'll feel the muscle bulging as you clench. When that occurs, your trigeminal nerve is firing.

Let's look at how your lower jaw can produce a migraine. Many of us grind or clench our teeth in very short intervals, five seconds or less, at night. You or your spouse may never notice it. That grinding puts the temporalis muscle into overdrive. The motor branch of the trigeminal nerve starts firing rapidly.

What do you think the activity of the motor branch of the trigeminal nerve does to the sensory branch of the trigeminal nerve? Yes. It causes the sensory branch to become active. Activity of the sensory branch increases the activity of the blood vessels. The blood vessels engorge, placing more pressure on the trigeminal sensory nerve. The result: a migraine.

You don't think you're grinding your teeth? Look in the mirror. Are some or all of your teeth flat? Even worse, are the edges of your teeth jagged? When you move your front teeth so that they are edge to edge, have you ground them so hard they fit together perfectly?

About 48 percent of migraines occur between 4 and 9 a.m. So, by the time you wake up, the migraine already is full-blown. It is difficult for medication to completely reverse such severe blood vessel inflammation, and the trigeminal nerve is already in a high state of electrical activity. It's difficult to control a fire when it is fully raging. It is more effective to prevent it. A simple dental appliance worn at night can reduce clenching and grinding, thus reducing muscle and trigeminal nerve activity. For many patients, such an appliance may make a significant improvement in the frequency and the severity of migraine headaches.

The Sinus Headache Myth

A PATIENT walks into my practice because she's heard that I know something about headaches. She's had lots of different treatments but no real success. She has what she describes as a "sinus headache." So I ask her if her sinuses feel blocked. She says that she can breathe fine. Has she seen a doctor to look at her sinuses? Yes, and the doctor says her sinuses are clear. "So how can it be a sinus headache?" I ask. "Well, I always feel my headaches under my cheekbones and behind my eyes," she answers.

The sinus is an air space. It is lined with a membrane and has various mechanisms for fluid to circulate around that membrane to keep it moist and clean. There are spaces and tubes for the fluid to drain. If those tubes are blocked, then the fluid becomes backed up, and you can have a true sinus headache. But let's be clear about something. What you feel as a "sinus headache" usually is not a sinus headache. It's a muscular headache. What difference does that make? It opens the way to an answer.

More often than not, the pain that you feel behind your eyes is actually coming from a "trigger point" in a muscle of the neck. In fact, this common trigger point not only causes pain behind the eye but also the back of the head, the top of the head, and behind the ear. Trigger points of the entire body were actually mapped out over sixty years ago by President Kennedy's physician, Dr. Janet Travell.

So here's what we did with the "sinus headache" patient. We applied ultrasound and cold laser and did manual muscle releases to the trigger points of the neck. And what do you think happened to her sinus headache? It was gone in less than an hour.

One single treatment will not cure this problem. After all, it took a long time for the muscles to develop their trigger points, and because the muscles of the head and neck all communicate with each other, they all need to be "untriggered" to stop her chronic headaches. In addition, the nerves of the neck and jaw muscles and the nerves of the teeth all communicate through the same nerve complex, the trigeminal nucleus. So as the muscles relax, we need to keep careful tabs on the jaw and teeth to make sure that they don't act as new triggers. It takes eight to twelve weeks for the triggered muscles to heal before a permanent improvement can occur.

With careful attention to relaxing the muscular triggers and monitoring the teeth to stop them from contributing to those triggers, you can have permanent improvement of not only sinus headaches, but most other headaches, including migraines.

The Chronic Headache: A Dental Answer

OVER 80 million of us in the United States suffer from chronic headaches, migraine, or TMJ/D issues according to the National Institutes of Health. That is more than one in four of every U.S. household. For most, it is a way of life. You wake up and it's another day of head pain. You take some pills to relieve the pain, but the pain is always there. It's just dulled a little bit. You have to function, so you try to block the pain out, find something productive to do so that you're not thinking about the pain. Every once in a while the pain becomes so severe that you can't even think of getting out of bed.

So you see the doctor. You have x-rays and scans done to rule out a brain tumor. And sure enough, you don't have a brain tumor. That's a relief! But still, the pain continues. You are given medication that you can take by mouth, maybe a medication that you can inject into your thigh when the pain becomes really bad, like a migraine. So you travel from moderate pain to occasional bouts of severe pain, but you never get any pain relief. In fact, it's been years since you had relief of pain. If you're nodding your head, you are this person, or you are very close to one who is this person.

So what does the chronic headache patient have in common with every other headache patient? First, you've probably had head trauma some time in your life. You may have gone to the emergency room, may have worn a cervical collar, probably were put on pain medications and muscle relaxants. It could have been caused by something small like a minor car accident years ago you have forgotten about or by something more memorable like having your wisdom teeth pulled. The question is did the head heal back in the same relative position, and the answer is likely not. The head has a myriad of nerves and muscles. It is connected to the rest of the body by the cervical vertebrae of the neck, and the head is connected to a bone that can swing right, left, up, and down. That is the jawbone. The jawbone is regulated by the position of the teeth, particularly when the mouth is closed. The teeth usually fit together just fine, like gears in a motor. But after head trauma, that fit may not be exactly the same; the gears are "off" a bit. The teeth have nerve receptors that send signals as to the proper position of things. So the teeth send out the signal that they are not in the correct relative position. This sends a message to other structures, such as the nerves, tendons, and muscles to put the jaw in the correct position. But the muscles, nerves, and tendons have to strain to do that. So now, instead of having a toothache, you have a jaw ache because the jaw is now out of position and the muscles are struggling to keep it in that position.

Those muscles can't hold that position very long without becoming tired and fatigued. They start to hurt, and because those muscles are connected to other muscles of the neck and the back of the head, they start to hurt, too.

It is actually the dentist that might produce the greatest improvement in this malady because the dentist can place a plastic jig in the mouth that, if prepared carefully, can short-circuit the nerve receptors, which can result in jaw relaxation.

Now, new technologies can assist in that treatment. Using a variety of modalities that measure the force of the bite on the teeth, we can better pinpoint the bite diagnosis. Through modalities often reserved for high-end sports medicine, a properly equipped and trained dentist can use microcurrent, ultrasound, and cold laser to rehabilitate the muscles. Once complete rehabilitation occurs, the bite can be lightly adjusted to recreate the normal dental forces within the normal jaw position.

So, if you have headaches, they could be dental-force related, and they don't have to remain. A simple, painless exam might answer the question. It is just a matter of reversing the trauma that put you in that position in the first place. With that accomplished, you can live a normal life again.

ORTHODONTICS

Braces at My Age?

REMEMBER being interested in how many cavities you had when you were young (or maybe not so interested)? Now you have weathered periodontal disease, worn teeth, crowns, bridges, partials, often losing some teeth along the way. So it's not the same as it was, and just as we need to remodel our houses at times from the bottom up, we sometimes have to rebuild our bites.

As we age, the importance of comprehensive treatment planning increases. Having the dentist fix one tooth at a time doesn't work as well as it did when we were younger because of the general deterioration that often occurs as the years pass.

In developing a comprehensive treatment plan, we often look at the changes that have occurred in tooth-to-tooth relationships. Teeth drift into spaces created by teeth that have been missing. So the teeth start to lean over. And just as the Leaning Tower of Pisa is not particularly stable, a slanted tooth may not be able to tolerate the generally vertical forces from chewing and the multiple forces that occur when we grind our teeth.

Sometimes teeth are never in the right position to begin with, but we live with it. The problem is that unfavorable tooth positions over time can result in loose teeth, and the body can no longer bounce back from or tolerate the adverse stresses being imposed on the teeth and underlying bone.

As we age, teeth often become more crowded, particularly in the front. People often ask me why their teeth are more crowded in the front at this stage of their lives than they were in the past. The answers are sometimes difficult to come by, but the fact is that teeth tend to move toward the center as we age, causing crowding that we never had when we were younger.

Therefore, an important part of a comprehensive dental treatment plan is to look at these factors and make sure that our teeth are in the best possible position in terms of appearance and function.

If teeth are out of alignment, the treatment is now easier and quicker than ever before. You've probably seen commercials for a technique that uses a series of clear plastic trays that move teeth without anyone even seeing that your teeth are being moved. And if traditional braces are desired, there is a periodontal surgical technique that can be used at the beginning of orthodontic treatment to make the treatment up to four times faster than traditional braces called "Periodontally Assisted Osteogenic Orthodontics."

The point is clear. Proper tooth alignment can help your teeth feel more comfortable and functional. Orthodontic tooth alignment is worth assessing as part of any full dental treatment plan.

Invisalign: Healthier, Straighter Teeth without Metal Braces

Matthew E. Sheldon, DMD

BRACES: A word for decades that meant you were a teenager with crooked teeth. Your parents would take you to the orthodontist, slap braces on your teeth for a couple of years, and give you a retainer that you would hopefully wear forever. Fortunately, times have changed, and technology has advanced. There is now a second option for most patients, not just teenagers, seeking straighter teeth without the unsightly metal brackets and wires, and that is Invisalign.

Studies have shown that 74 person of American adults have malocclusion. That means 3 out of every 4 of us have a bite that isn't ideal. A bad bite can lead to numerous problems down the road. The first is dental hygiene. It's just that much more difficult to take care of crooked teeth. Bacteria accumulate in unreachable nooks and crannies. Some of those bacteria smell. Guess where that smell goes.

The next problem that a bad bite can lead to is wear and trauma to your teeth. Teeth are made to fit evenly. The upper front teeth should overlap the lower front teeth a bit. The whole system of teeth is made to gently guide your jaw when chewing, but teeth that aren't straight create extra stress and pressure on your teeth. If the system doesn't work correctly, the result is chipped teeth, notches in your teeth at the gum line called abfractions, premature wear, and even mobility of the teeth.

So what is Invisalign, and how is it different? Invisalign is a series of clear plastic trays that you wear all the time, except when you eat or drink anything besides water. We take digital impressions and photographs, and in a matter of weeks, treatment can begin. The wonderful thing about taking digital impressions with Invisalign is that the software can simulate what your teeth will look like at the end of treatment. That means that right after we take the digital impressions, you can see on the screen what your teeth will look like after treatment. Each set of trays is worn for two weeks. Then you move on to the next set, gradually moving your teeth in the correct direction. You will generally see your Invisalign dentist every six weeks to make sure things are moving properly. Occasionally, you may need some teeth adjusted to make them a bit narrower to eliminate crowding. You may also need a small adhesive button on one or more of your teeth. The trays grab on to this clear button to help facilitate the movement of a tooth more quickly.

The only problem that I have seen with any removable clear-tray system like Invisalign is that you have the option to choose when you wear the trays since they are removable. You need to wear the trays at least twenty-one hours a day for the system to work. If you wear them less than that, your next set of trays won't fit properly, and that will cause a delay in treatment.

I was my very first Invisalign patient. I knew I wanted straight teeth since high school but didn't want to wear braces years after my friends were out of braces. My problem was spaces between most of my front teeth. I flossed and brushed twice a day, but my gums were still always tender and would bleed during my regularly scheduled cleanings. During treatment, my patients wouldn't believe I was wearing Invisalign trays until I showed it to them up close. Since completing treatment, my teeth are straighter and noticeably healthier. Food doesn't get lodged anymore, and my gums have never felt better. I get complimented on my straight teeth all the time, something I never heard before when I had the gaps in my teeth.

The Periodontist and Orthodontist Combine Forces

ORTHODONTIC treatment (Braces) can help both children and adults smile and chew better. Two former problems have now been solved by combining the disciplines of periodontics and orthodontics.

One barrier is time. Traditional orthodontic treatment takes up to two years or even longer. To simplify the discussion, let's think of a specialized ship, an ice breaker, going through the frozen southern Atlantic Ocean. The ice breaker needs to move at a deliberately slow speed to open the waterway without damaging the ship. If it goes too fast, the ice may not break down fast enough to allow passage of the ship or even worse, may cause damage to the hull. The same concept applies to orthodontic treatment. Treatment can't be rushed as too much orthodontic pressure may cause damage to the root surfaces as they are being moved through the bone. And the harder the bone, the slower the teeth move.

The second barrier is "thin bone," described previously in this book. Now teeth may move very quickly through thin bone, but if the tooth is moved out of the bone support, there is an increased likelihood of pressure on the gums and consequent gum recession.

So how do we solve these seemingly unsolvable problems? Can we make the hard bone softer so that the teeth will move faster? Can we increase the width of thin bone to allow the teeth to be moved to their proper position without damaging the gums? The answer is Yes. And both seemingly opposite problems can be solved with the same procedure, Periodontally Assisted Osteogenic Orthodontics or PAOO.

Here's how PAOO works. The gums tissues are surgically peeled away from the underlying bone. A very small dental drill is used to make small holes through the surface cortex of the bone. This then causes the bone to begin the healing process, which begins with localized inflammation. What happens during inflammation? The body sends cells called osteoclasts to take away the bone damaged by the small holes. This causes the bone to temporarily soften. To use the previous analogy, the ice melts.The body then sends new bone-forming cells called osteoblasts to the area to heal the bone. The new bone calcifies and within a few months, hardens back to the original state. But during the time that the bone is soft, the teeth can be moved faster without damaging them. In fact, a PAOO case can go four times faster than traditional orthodontics alone.

But wait, you say. I understand how PAOO can increase orthodontic speed, but what about the thin bone? Now I'll add the final piece to PAOO. We do bone grafts at the same time as we make the small holes. The bone grafts consist of a powder that's placed over the existing bone. That powder becomes bone over time. So with the bone grafts the thin bone case becomes thicker. The teeth can be moved into their proper position because there is new bone toward which the teeth can be moved.

PAOO has been researched and continues to be researched in the university setting. It's been done clinically for over 15 years. What is clear from x rays and CT scans of completed cases is that orthodontic treatment can now take as little as 4-6 months with PAOO, providing additional bone support with less root damage than the traditional approach.

Why Recession? Why Crowding? And Why Impacted Teeth (Especially Wisdom Teeth)?

Colin Richman, DMD

"IT do so many people have impacted wisdom teeth," you might ask. You might as well add two other questions to the mix. Why are the gums so thin on the lower front teeth, and why are the lower front teeth crowded so often? Half of us in the United States have one or more of these three conditions. I was puzzled by this as well, and no one had done research to answer those questions. I see a lot of patients with these conditions and have seen or done lots of gum tissue grafts, orthodontic treatment, and extraction of wisdom teeth. One advantage I have is that I have CT scans on many of my patients, so I have a good database from which to study these issues.

What I have found is that the three conditions—impacted wisdom teeth, gum recession, and tooth crowding—are related to each other. The name that I've given it is Dental Space Deficiency Syndrome (DSDS). As I reviewed not only my CT scan data but also data from anthropologists who have studied skulls from thousands of years ago, I made some observations.

The first observation is that our jaws are slowly decreasing in size. Why might this occur? All we have to do is study the lifestyles of prehistoric man against our current lifestyles to derive an answer. Prehistoric men were hunters and gatherers. Later, farming became the primary way of providing food. And now—well you know what we do now, with cooked and soft processed food, microwaved food, and the like. So as man developed, there was less and less work for the jaw to do, so it has become smaller and smaller. Our jaw size has changed because of the function required of it.

But tooth size is not determined by function. It is determined by genetics. So as our jaws are getting smaller and smaller, our teeth are staying the same size. The result? There is not as much room for the teeth, so they are impacted, crowded, and have gum recession.

We do have some answers to DSDS. Orthodontists can move teeth to create more bone, but there are limitations. If the jaw bone is narrower than the root of the tooth and we try to widen the jaw with braces, the tooth may move through the bone, causing recession. How do we evaluate that in advance? A CT scan shows us the three-dimensional relationship of the tooth to the bone and can help us with that prediction. If we see that the bone is too narrow, we can do a bone graft in conjunction with braces, creating a larger volume of bone within which to move the tooth. There are additional advantages to this as the teeth will move faster and the chance of gum recession will be reduced.

Of course, oral surgeons help us by removing the wisdom teeth that we no longer have room for. If there is gum recession, periodontists have numerous tools at their disposal to add gum tissue and bone tissue as necessary. Where do we get the bone. Usually from a bone bank that has created bone for this purpose. And the gum? We have tissue banks for that. Sometimes we need to go to the palate for the best gum tissue, but even that procedure is improved with small incisions that spare the top layer of the gum tissue of the palate, making that area of the roof of the mouth quite comfortable after surgery. Dr. Sheldon speaks about treatment of gum recession elsewhere in this book.

Other conditions associated with DSDS include sleep apnea because the tongue is constricted by the reduced jaw bone. This can have ramifications even as children are developing. Constricted space means that more genetically determined organs are crammed into a smaller area.

There is one other thing to consider. If you have teeth extracted, limited bone may mean limited volume of bone after healing, so a bone graft after extraction, which is quite simple to do, may be essential, particularly if you are getting dental implants or if you want to maintain the cosmetics of the gum tissue that is supported by that bone.

Here are some cases that illustrate the problem of DSDS. The key is to get a diagnosis as soon as you see crowding, impacted wisdom teeth, or gum recession. With proper care, we can harness your jaw bone and your gum tissue to create an environment of life-long cosmetics and function.

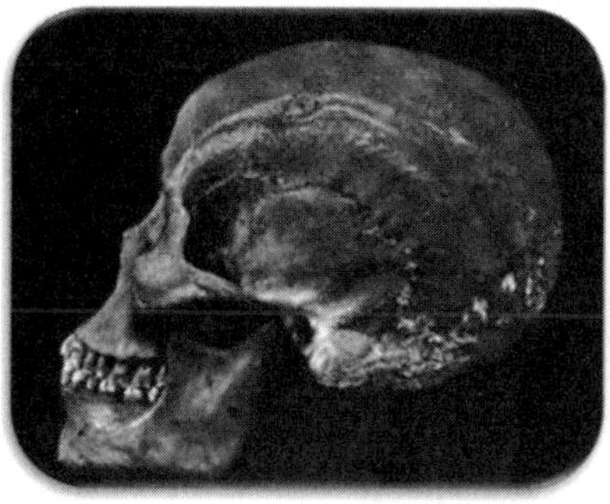

Skull of prehistoric man

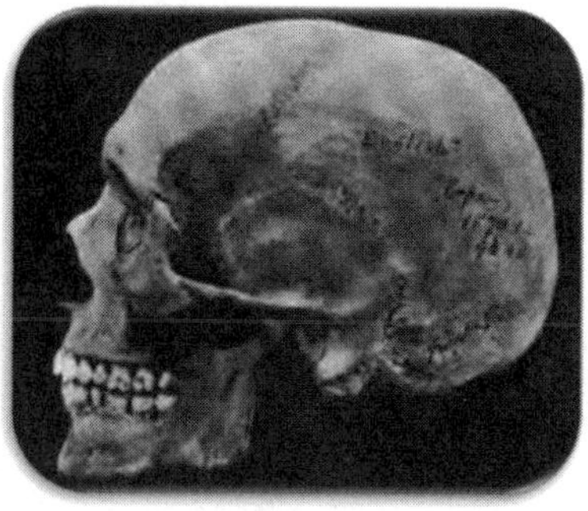

Skull of modern man

The following two cases illustrate the DSDS condition.

Case 1—Eight-year-old

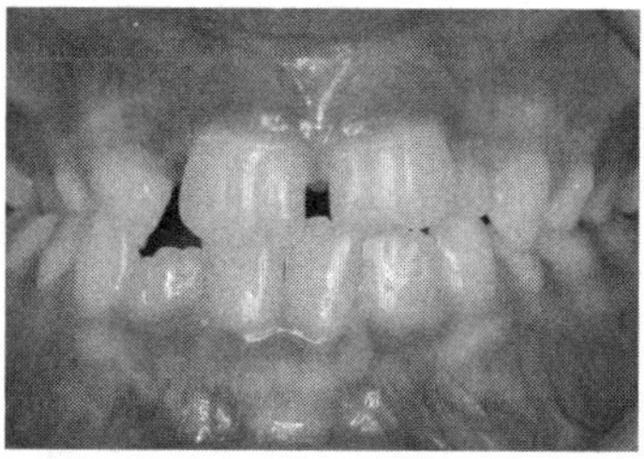

Ultra thin gingival (gum) tissue with early recession of lower teeth

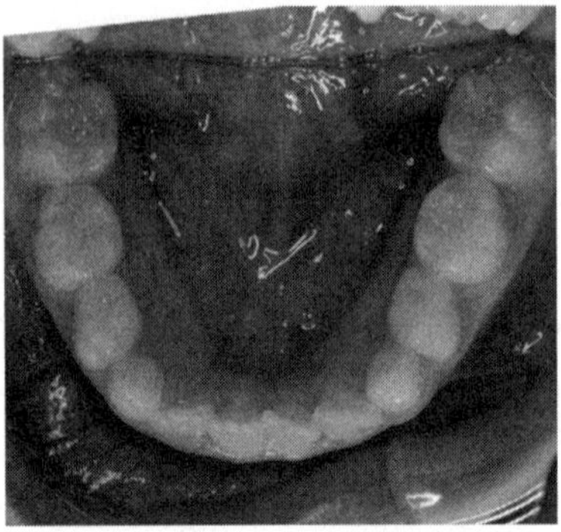

Crowded permanent teeth in this eight-year-old patient with insufficient jaw bone space to accommodate the permanent teeth

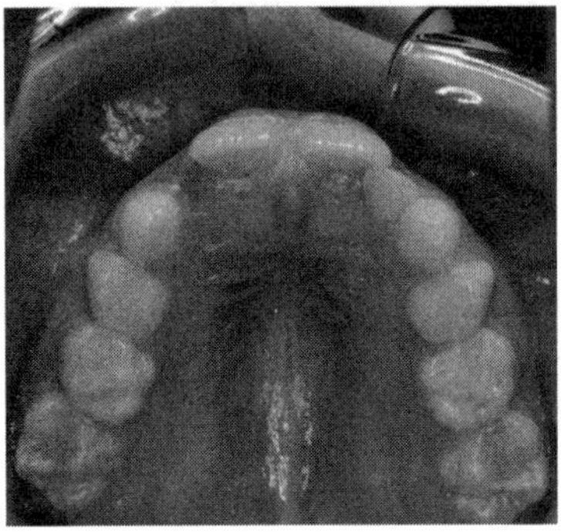

Crowded front (deciduous) teeth

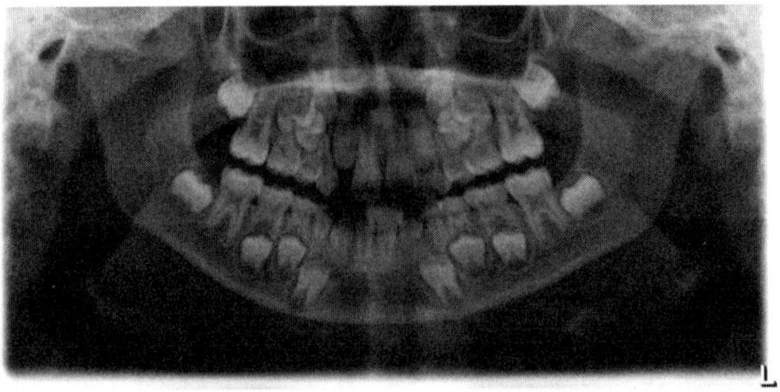

Panoramic radiograph showing crowded teeth with insufficient space for permanent teeth

Case 2—Permanent dentition

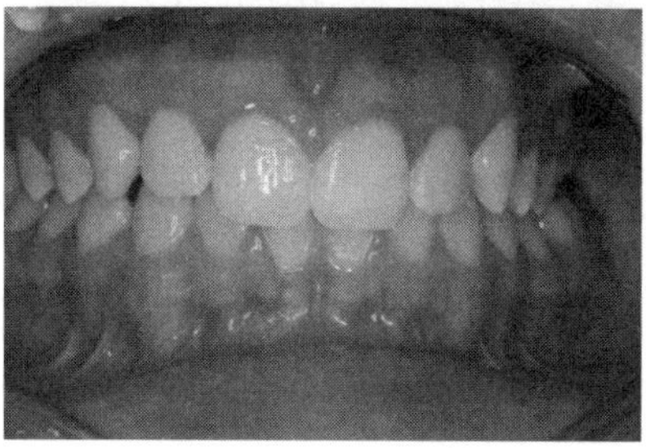

Adult patient, thin gum tissue, gum recession of lower front teeth and upper left canine

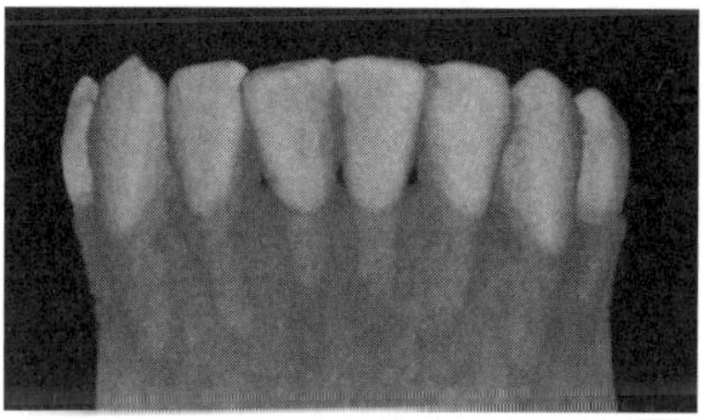

Same patient, CT scan demonstrating ultra-thin bone covering the roots of the lower jaw teeth, rendering these teeth at future risk for gum recession

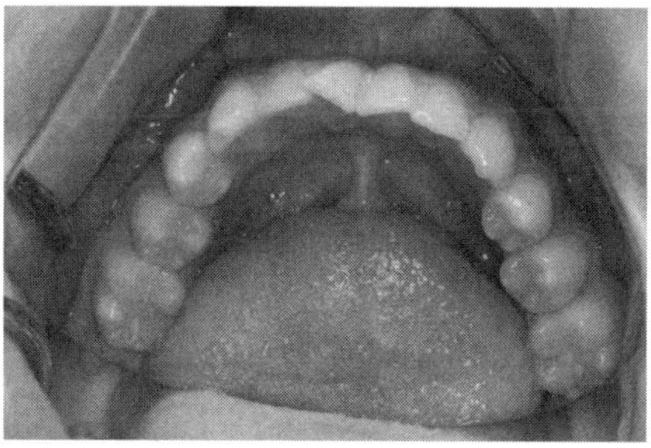

Crowded lower front teeth (DSDS)

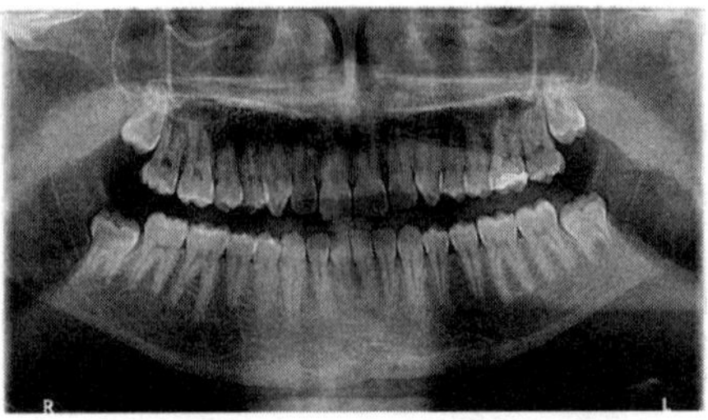

Panoramic radiograph demonstrating impacted third molars (wisdom teeth) due to inadequate jaw bone space available to accommodate these teeth

Dr. Colin Richman practices periodontics and implant dentistry in Roswell, Georgia. He is Assistant Clinical Professor in the Department of Periodontics at Medical College of Georgia, Georgia Regents University. His website is www.drcolinrichman.com.

SLEEP APNEA

Addressing Obstructive Sleep Apnea is Vital to Your Health

IT isn't just snoring. People snore. It is a normal life occurrence, isn't it? When people snore it becomes a problem—more for the bed partner than the snorer him or herself.

If snoring were the only problem, then it would be considered to be a mere nuisance, and frankly it was considered only a nuisance until recently. It is only recently that we found out that snoring actually becomes a much more severe problem, one that increases the risk of some very life-threatening diseases. Heart attack and stroke are first that come to mind, and recently diabetes and hypercholesterolemia (too much cholesterol in the blood) have been added to the list. In other words, the stopping of breathing that occurs when you snore, which is what sleep apnea is all about, increases the risk of experiencing life-threatening events.

It happens simply. It happens slowly. It takes a while for a person to go from being a mild snorer to a moderate snorer, to a severe snorer, and finally to developing sleep apnea. What we find is that most people don't know they have sleep apnea. I didn't! The only way I found out was by having a sleep test called a polysomnogram, which revealed just how significant the problem was for me.

We are fortunate in our county to have several competent sleep physicians. I have gotten to know them. I have been in a sleep lab. I see how comfortable a sleep lab is, and while you think you don't want to go to sleep with a lot of wires attached to you, these sleep labs have become so comfortable that it is like being in a hotel room. If you have any doubt as to whether a test in a sleep lab is valid, there are scientific studies to prove that. Now we aren't subjects of scientific studies. We are people who are suffering from something that we don't think is going to cause us a problem. The fact is, a sleep lab will determine for us whether it is a problem or not.

Once an Obstructive Sleep Apnea diagnosis is made, then you have a choice as to how you want to be treated. The CPAP (Continuous Positive Airway Pressure) is the most reliable form of treatment. Unfortunately, only about 50% of the people who use CPAP like it, and that's why we have spent a lot of time developing expertise and developing intraoral appliances which open the airway. The appliances do not work quite as well or quite as predictably as CPAP, but they work predictably enough to make them a very strong first alternative to CPAP, according to the American Academy of Sleep Medicine.

The first thing to do is get a diagnosis. Go see a sleep physician. I have recommended lots of people to sleep physicians. The diagnosis is thorough. People do better as a result. They sound better. They don't snore any more.

So if this chapter will only get you to a sleep physician, you've come a long way. If you have already seen a sleep physician, and CPAP doesn't work for you, then certainly an oral appliance should be very high on your priority list.

So how do you know that you have a sleep problem. One test that is commonly used is the Epworth Sleepiness Scale. It's a standard test used in many sleep physicians' offices. So let's see how you score.

Epworth Sleepiness Scale

The Epworth Sleepiness Scale is used to determine the level of daytime sleepiness. A score of 10 or more is considered sleepy. A score of 18 or more is very sleepy. If you score 10 or more on this test, you should consider whether you are obtaining adequate sleep, need to improve your sleep hygiene and/or need to see a sleep specialist. These issues should be discussed with your personal physician.

Use the following scale to choose the most appropriate number for each situation:

0 = would *never* doze or sleep.
1 = *slight* chance of dozing or sleeping
2 = *moderate* chance of dozing or sleeping
3 = *high* chance of dozing or sleeping

Fill in your answers and see where you stand.

Situation	Chance of Dozing or Sleeping
Sitting and reading	___
Watching TV	___
Sitting inactive in a public place	___
Being a passenger in a motor vehicle for an hour or more	___
Lying down in the afternoon	___
Sitting and talking to someone	___
Sitting quietly after lunch (no alcohol)	___
Stopped for a few minutes in traffic while driving	___
Total score (add the scores up) (This is your Epworth score)	___

This questionnaire from the University of Maryland may help you even further.

Questionnaire for Sleep Apnea Risk

Assess your risk for sleep apnea. The total score for all 5 sections is your *Apnea Risk Score*. Print out this questionnaire, write in your best answer for each question and see where you stand.

A. How frequently do you experience or have you been told about snoring loud enough to disturb the sleep of others?
   1. Never
   2. Rarely (less than once a week)
   3. Occasionally (1 - 3 times a week)
   4. Frequently (More than 3 times a week)

   Answer_____

B. How often have you been told that you have "pauses" in breathing or stop breathing during sleep?
   1. Never
   2. Rarely (less than once a week)
   3. Occasionally (1 - 3 times a week)
   4. Frequently (More than 3 times a week)

   Answer_____

C. How much are you overweight?
   1. Not at all
   2. Slightly (10 - 20 pounds)
   3. Moderately (20 - 40 pounds)
   4. Severely (More than 40 pounds)

   Answer______

D. What is your Epworth Sleepiness Score?
   1. Less than 8
   2. 9 -13
   3. 14 - 18
   4. 19 or greater

   Answer ______

E. Does your medical history include:
   1. High blood pressure
   2. Stroke
   3. Heart disease
   4. More than 3 awakenings per night (on the average)
   5. Excessive fatigue
   6. Difficulty concentrating or staying awake during the day

   Answer ______

If you answered 3) or 4) for questions A-D, especially if you have one or more of the conditions listed in question E, then you may be at risk for sleep apnea and should discuss this with your physician.

Note: You should always discuss sleep-related complaints with your physician before deciding on medical evaluation and treatment.

Can't Wear a CPAP Mask? Your Dentist May Be Able to Help

OBSTRUCTIVE sleep apnea (OSA) is a chronic condition when it causes disturbances in sleep three or more nights a week. It occurs in males twice as often as in females. As we age, we lose muscle tonus in many areas of the body, including the mouth and throat. Just as you may be a little flabby in your belly, you also become flabby in the muscles controlling your airway. The usual scenario is this: You fall asleep on your back. Your tongue falls back toward your throat. Your soft palate and your pharynx also collapse a bit. You start to snore as the air that you inhale goes through the airway, which is now narrowed because of the muscle collapse. What happens if those airway muscles completely collapse? You stop breathing. Of course, you won't let your body do this for too long, so you wake up just enough to tighten the muscles in your airway and start breathing again.

This process can occur several times per hour. The more often you are awakened out of a deep sleep, the more tired you're likely to be the next day, but it doesn't stop there. OSA increases the risk of high blood pressure, heart attack, stroke, obesity, and diabetes.

The first-line treatment for OSA is CPAP (Continuous Positive Airway Pressure), a nasal and/or oral mask connected by hose to a machine that blows air into your airway to keep it from collapsing. Despite its effectiveness, many with OSA, particularly in a mild or moderate form, find the CPAP to be a nuisance and don't use it. Or they find it so confining that they cannot wear the mask.

The next alternative to CPAP, according to the American Academy of Sleep Medicine, it is an oral appliance. This device, worn on top of the teeth, opens your jaw and moves it forward, thus opening your airway.

You can try it yourself. Take a deep breath through your mouth and feel the air going through the airway. Now thrust your lower jaw forward and take another deep breath. Do you feel a difference? You've just opened your airway. The oral appliance opens the airway in the same fashion, stopping snoring and alleviating obstructive sleep apnea for many. It is the most predictable solution for those who don't like CPAP.

There are many oral appliances available for OSA. The best are adjustable appliances that allow you or your dentist to put your jaw in the most ideal position to open your airway. The use of such an appliance may not only make you a less noisy bed partner, it may also save you from daytime fatigue as well as reduce your risk of some serious diseases.

OVERALL HEALTH CARE

Recurrent Mouth Sores

YOU feel a small, sore area on the inside of your lip or tongue. It wasn't there yesterday. It just showed up. You have a canker sore or, in our terms, an aphthous ulcer. They are usually less than a 1/2 inch in diameter, oval, and have a red border and a whitish or yellowish center. You'll sometimes feel a tingling sensation in the area for a couple of days before they actually show up.

Don't confuse a canker sore with a cold sore. Cold sores are from viruses and are usually found on the dry portion of the lip or on hard surfaces in the mouth, such as the palate. Cold sores are from the Herpes virus, are contagious, and respond to anti-viral medications. Canker sores occur on the loose, wet tissue of the inner lips, below the gum line, and under the tongue. They are neither viral nor contagious.

What causes canker sores? Most often, they just appear for no reason. However, they can be caused by rough edges on your teeth, sensitivities to foods, particularly chocolate (Sorry!), coffee, strawberries, eggs, nuts, cheese, as well as highly acidic foods. They can be related to food allergies as well as a diet lacking in vitamin B12, zinc, folate, and iron. Canker sores can also be caused by Helicobacter pylori, the same bacteria that cause stomach ulcers, and can be related to gluten sensitivities and inflammatory bowel diseases. Occasionally, I'll see a patient whose canker sores clear up just by their changing toothpastes away from those that have the additive Sodium Lauryl Sulfate. Canker sores are genetically related about a third of the time.

One key to our helping you is by obtaining your diet and medication history. When did the canker sores start? What were you eating? Have there been recent changes in your diet? Have you started taking a new medication?

While canker sores are a nuisance, they're usually not dangerous. If they are large or if you often get clusters of them, it would be worthwhile to get some blood tests and maybe a biopsy, but that's the rare exception.

What are the treatments? The best treatment is no treatment. They'll usually go away by themselves. If they are a nuisance, then your dentist or physician can prescribe antibacterial mouth rinses, topical pastes, and sometimes drugs that are used for heartburn or gout, and even cortisone preparations. There is a topical solution called Debacterol that your dentist or physician can paint on the sore to cauterize it. Nutritional supplements can also be prescribed. I even had one patient with the most severe canker sores for years completely clear up after one chiropractic adjustment.

The key is that if canker sores are just now showing up, look at the changes that you've made in your medications. Usually, you can be the best detective in determining why they started. Your doctor can then help you find an alternative.

Let's Start Taking Control of Our Health

WE ARE OVERMEDICATED!

YES, I know that your doctor said that you have osteopenia, high cholesterol, diabetes, high blood pressure, etc., etc. It's not the diagnosis that I doubt. Your doctor examined you and found the problems. That is *diagnosis.*

It is the *treatment* that is the problem.

Let's go back to a time when prescription medications were never advertised. Let's go back to a time when you saw your doctor for advice, not for a prescription. It wasn't that long ago, was it? And let's stop fooling ourselves. Our bodies are not much different from similar people 50 years ago, except for the fact that we eat more, ingest more processed foods, drink more, and take more medications. We eat more junk food, fast food, more snacks, and more sugar, which makes us eat even more sugar. And that's not the way our grandparents ate. We sleep less, spend less time with our families, more time on the internet, less time at church, at clubs, etc., etc. Our bodies are the same bodies as those of our grandparents, but our lifestyles are not.

So here's what we do. We see the doctor and get a prescription. The doctor tells us to come back and see him/her in three months. We see the numbers on our blood test go down, and we cheer. What's to cheer about? The medication makes our numbers look okay, but are we really okay?

Even worse, a medication creates side effects, which may require another medication. So we get that prescription, and we temporarily feel better. The medication is safe. After all, it was approved by the FDA. Guess what? Those two medications were never tested together. They were only tested individually. And the problem magnifies when you take a third drug, and a fourth. I've seen patients who were taking over 20 different medications.

The answer is simpler than you think. When your doctor makes a diagnosis, listen to the diagnosis. You may need a medication. But then you have a job to do. That job is to find all the ways in which you created the diagnosis to begin with and fix that, so that you can get off of the medication. And when you tell your doctor that's what you'd like to do, he or she will monitor your progress. Sound impossible? I have been to two wellness clinics, and I have seen some of the sickest people you can imagine, under doctors' supervision, get off of all, or nearly all, of their medications. Their tests normalize. They feel better than they have in years.

Please take control of your health. Start reading. Start planning; look for answers. They are not hard to find. Make the commitment to changing yourself. If you want a list of newsletters that I recommend, please email me at LeeNSheldon@cfl.rr.com or call my office. You can start the process of regaining your health.

Do You Really Need That Pill?

THERE are times when we look at something, and it's more comfortable to turn away. After all, confronting something is difficult. It's often much easier to go with the flow. But the flow brings us downstream. That's where the muck and the silt is. It's the path of least resistance. And it often leads to failure.

So where are we failing? We are failing in health care. I'm not going to play the Obamacare game. That's for someone much more politically astute than I am. But the fact that we are even debating Obamacare is the problem. We can debate insurance, we can debate Medicare, we can debate how big the safety net should be, we can even debate who should pay for what and whether health care is a right or a privilege.

But we can't debate personal responsibility. We can't debate our own personal responsibility for our health. There's some feeling that we've acquired that we need pills, that we need medications not to survive, but to prevent a problem. We take anti-cholesterol pills, anti osteoporosis pills, anti behavior disorder pills, anti blood pressure pills, anti-diabetes pills. We ask the pills to stop something, but we have no regard for the other things that those pills stop. We say that this is health care. And you know what? It's not.

What it is, is satisfying ourselves that because certain blood tests say we are abnormal, we then take a pill. And then when the tests are "normal" again, that we are healthy. Well, guess what! That's not true! We take the first pill. Then because of a side effect of that pill, we take another, and another, and another. In the meantime, we don't pay enough attention to what we can and should do for our health; simple things like eating enough fruits and vegetables. We lose the importance of that. We lose the importance of the nutrition that will make us far healthier than a "prevention pill" will ever make us. We think that because our overworked doctors recommend the pill, that's the only way. But here's the rub. The healthiest doctors don't take all those pills. They're at the gym. They're eating good foods. They're reading to find out what they can do better to maintain their health. And unless it's a life-threatening condition, they are trying everything to prevent themselves from having to take pills.

Somehow, we've gotten the idea that we can't know enough to make health care decisions. It's funny. When you're in my office and have to make a decision, you ask me the benefits, the risks, and how much it will cost. When your doctor makes a recommendation, how often do you ask him or her the same things? Often, when it's paid for by someone else, we somehow take less interest in the subject.

I will tell you a fact. You can make your own health care decisions. You can read. You can educate yourself. You can reverse the course of nearly every disease. And certainly you can prevent most diseases without pills. It's a running theme in our office. When I look at you, I'm not just looking at your teeth, your gums, your bone, your headaches. I'm looking at you, all of you. I'm looking at what you can do better. Some of you have made miraculous changes in your health by taking more responsibility for what goes into your bodies and what doesn't. And when you do, not only will your oral health be better, so will your general health.

Your Responsibility for Your Health Is Yours

THERE are times when we look at something and it's more comfortable to turn away. After all, confronting something is difficult. It's often much easier to go with the flow, but the flow brings us downstream. That's where the muck and the silt is. It's the path of least resistance, and it often leads to failure.

So where are we failing? We are failing in health care. I'm not going to play the Obamacare game. That's for someone much more politically astute than I am. But the fact that we are even debating Obamacare as the focus of health care is the problem. We can debate insurance, we can debate Medicare, we can debate how big the safety net should be, we can even debate who should pay for what and whether health care is a right or a privilege, but we can't debate personal responsibility. We can't debate our own personal responsibility for our health. There's some feeling that we've acquired that we need pills, that we need medications not to survive, but to prevent a problem. We take anti-cholesterol pills, anti-osteoporosis pills, anti-behavior disorder pills, anti-blood pressure pills, anti-diabetes pills. We ask the pills to stop something, but we have no regard for the other things that those pills stop. We say that this is health care, but you know what? It's not.

What it is, is satisfying ourselves that because certain blood tests say we are abnormal, we then take a pill, and then when the tests are "normal" again, we say we are healthy. Well, guess what? That's not true! We take the first pill. Then because of a side effect of that pill, we take another, and another, and another. In the meantime, we don't pay enough attention to what we can and should do for our health—simple things like eating enough fruits and vegetables, simple things like avoiding processed foods. We lose the importance of that. We lose the importance of the nutrition that will make us far healthier than a "prevention pill" will ever make us. We think that because our overworked doctors recommend the pill, that's the only way. But here's the rub: the healthiest doctors don't take all those pills. They're at the gym. They're eating good foods. They're reading to find out what they can do better to maintain their health, and unless it's a life-threatening condition, they are trying everything to prevent themselves from having to take pills.

Somehow, we've gotten the idea that we can't know enough to make health care decisions. It's funny. When you're in the dental office and have to make a decision, you ask the benefits, the risks, and how much it will cost. You ask about alternatives. When your doctor makes a recommendation, how often do you ask him or her the same things? Often, when it's paid for by someone else, we somehow take less interest in the subject.

I will tell you a fact: you can make your own health care decisions. You can read. You can educate yourself. You can reverse the course of nearly every disease, and certainly you can prevent most diseases without pills. I've seen it in my own patients. When I look at them, I'm not just looking at their teeth, their gums, their bones, their facial muscles, their headaches, or their sleep apnea. I'm looking at them, period. I'm not alone.

We in the health professions are looking at you from our own particular viewpoints. We look not only at disease; we look at what you can do better. Some of you have made miraculous changes in your health by taking more responsibility for what goes into your bodies and what doesn't, what you choose to do and what you don't, and when you take that level of responsibility, not only will your oral health be better, so will your general health.

A Different Approach to Chronic Disease

HAVE you thought that you want to change the course of your health care? Are you taking more and more medications and want to get off of them and improve your health? Do you want to take a comprehensive approach to really get back to health again?

As I write this, I am at such a wellness center. People come here from all over the country to regain their health. I am fortunate in that my problems are minor by comparison with most that are here. Most are here with serious heart disease and diabetes. Many others are here with chronic pain, chronic respiratory problems, neurologic problems, or chronic fatigue, or they are interested in anti-aging therapies. They just want to feel better.

The sequence followed is this: On my first day, I am examined by my physician. He spends at least an hour with his new patients, just getting history and your goals for your time here. Blood and other tests are done on the first day. Based upon your symptoms, an initial program is prescribed for you. Some of the therapies include intravenous nutrients, hyperbaric oxygen therapy, reflexology, massage, and acupuncture. Some of the unique therapies include EECP (enhanced external counterpulsation), a system developed at Harvard that produces new blood vessels around clogged arteries. Many with angina and who want an alternative to bypass surgery use EECP. Other therapies include microcurrent and infrared light therapies for relief of chronic pain, high-intensity laser therapy for relief of joint conditions, and bioidentical hormone therapy to reduce the effects of aging. The list of therapies is too long to recite in this column.

The point is this: there are successful, non-pharmacologic therapies available. In a comprehensive facility, you have the opportunity to be supervised by a physician and subjectively and objectively evaluate your success. Once you and your physician evaluate which therapies are most successful for you, you are then given a program to take home where you may continue those therapies. As many of the therapies are available from multiple healers in Brevard county, you can continue your successful treatment here. Your local physician can help you in monitoring the success of such treatment, and you can be in phone consultation with the original wellness center physician as well.

One question always asked is whether such evaluation and treatment is covered by insurance. Some is, but likely most is not. The people that I meet at these centers are not all well-to-do, but they have decided to use their own personal resources to take advantage of the health benefits provided by this and other centers throughout the country.

[The material in this column is for informational purposes only. You should consult with your physician before making any changes in your health care regimen.]

If you feel that you are on a path of taking more and more medications and feeling and doing worse, there are other answers out there. With a little research on your part, you may find the perfect answer for you.

Three Good Reasons to See a Dentist BEFORE Receiving Cancer Treatment

YOU'VE received the news. You or a loved one needs to be treated for cancer. Now you go through the process of thinking about the treatment and the changes that you may need to make to be sure that the treatment is most effective. That may involve lifestyle and dietary improvements as well as the cancer treatment itself. One area that is often neglected but should be addressed early is the health of your mouth.

The National Institute of Health lists three reasons to see the dentist before cancer treatment.

1. You'll feel better.
2. You'll help protect your teeth, gums, and bone.
3. You'll prevent needless delays and complications that can occur if oral infections occur after cancer treatment.

In addition to surgery, the two primary treatments for cancer are radiation and chemotherapy. Let's look at radiation first. Radiation to the head and neck area has two potentially devastating side effects.

1. **Radiation to the head and neck kills the salivary glands in its field, producing a dry mouth.** When the mouth is dry, it becomes acidic. And an acidic mouth becomes prone to dental decay. Therefore, all decay should be diagnosed and treated before radiation therapy. In addition, a preventive protocol that might include fluoride, xylitol (sugar that helps stop tooth decay), baking soda rinses, and artificial salivas might be prescribed to help prevent decay. Intensive home care can

prevent decay and the potential of tooth loss. Tooth extraction after radiation can be devastating because…

2. **Radiation to the head and neck reduces the blood supply to the bone and soft tissues.** If an extraction is necessary after radiation, there are increased complications from infection as the blood supply to the area is compromised. It is much less risky to have a tooth extracted before radiation therapy than afterward.

Chemotherapy has a much more generalized effect as it usually permeates the entire body. Side effects include soreness or ulcerations of the soft tissue of your mouth, dry mouth, a burning, peeling, or swelling tongue, infection, and taste changes. Oral rinses that numb the mouth may help you get through this period.

If I were diagnosed with cancer, I would get to a dentist immediately. Your dentist and oncologist will communicate with one another and coordinate efforts to reduce your risk during treatment. If an extraction is necessary, get it done as soon as possible before chemotherapy or radiation as adequate healing time of the extraction site is necessary before beginning radiation or chemotherapy. And your dentist will get you on a protocol to help keep you as comfortable as possible and reduce future risk of dental disease. Even if you never did it before, this is the time to keep up regular dental visits where prevention is emphasized and early diagnosis could be critical. Dental examination and treatment is a step that should not be overlooked as part of overall cancer therapy.

Sugar

WHEN was the last time you went to the store, or to the bakery, or to the restaurant and lulled yourself into that tasty "low fat" dessert. After all, you said it's low fat. It must be good for me. If only that were true. If the label says "low fat," beware! It means that it has to be high in something else, right? I know. They don't tell you that part. What do you think that food is high in? It's sugar—yes, pure, adulterated sugar.

Here are some basics: If it's processed, it's not very good for you. "Processed" means that the food has hit a machine before it got to you, so if it's in a can or, particularly, a box, it's processed. And if it's processed, the processing machine ate the good stuff and gave you sugar, sodium, and enough preservatives for the product to last long enough on the shelf that you can buy and store it.

Sugar comes in many different forms, and if it has -ose, as in sucrose, dextrose, and fructose, it's sugar. There are other sugars that don't have -ose, such as turbinado, maltodextrin, honey, and corn syrup.

It's funny how things have changed. We know that sugar is bad for us. We know we're not supposed to eat it. Now we have a new bad guy, high-fructose corn syrup, which may be even worse than traditional sugar. Now we're (I'm) searching for products with "real sugar," treating that sugar almost as a health food. How silly! What a change in our standards in only a generation.

Someone told me that we need to eat sugar "in moderation." I suppose that's true, except for the fact that our definition of "moderation" has changed so much in such a short period of time. Moderation in our parents' and grandparents' times was a trip to a fast-food joint once a month. They would bake fresh cookies that would last a few days. What's the definition of moderation now? Do you think our bodies and their ability to assimilate lots of junk food have changed in such a short period of time? Of course not!

Sugar is made to be used quickly. It is easily digested into glucose, which is used by the muscles to provide quick energy. However, if you don't use those muscles, if you don't exercise right away, the sugar doesn't just disappear. The liver has to handle it, and it turns the sugar into triglycerides, a component of fat. Triglycerides are directly related to cardiovascular disease, inflammation, diabetes, and a host of chronic degenerative diseases.

We'll talk about the danger of triglycerides in the next chapter. In the meantime, do something good for yourself besides forgoing sugar. Order a good health newsletter. My material for this chapter comes from one of my favorites, *Alternatives,* by Dr. David Williams. You can order it at drdavidwilliams.com or call 800-219-8591.

It's Not Just Fat and Cholesterol

CAN your liver deliver? When was the last time you saw an ad that emphasized your liver? We don't even serve liver and onions any more. The poor, ignored liver; it sits there as the ultimate filter for the bad things we eat, it makes cholesterol, it stores some vitamins, produces substances that break down fats, and converts blood glucose into glycogen so that it can store the carbohydrates that we eat, and it converts sugar into triglycerides. It's that sugar to triglyceride conversion that we're going to concentrate on, because it is what is causing us to be FAT.

"Right," you say sarcastically. "I never heard that. I'm on a low-fat diet, I use fat-blockers, I buy low-fat eggs, ice cream, yogurt, cakes, cookies, pies, etc., etc." Boy, have we been sold a bill of goods. Now do you really think that something that is called "low-fat" really creates low fat? We're buying a lot of "low fat" products. And I hear that the scale near the doorway of Publix is calling for reinforcements.

So here's what happens when you eat "low-fat." Unless you're eating cardboard, (even rice cakes are high in sugar) you're eating high sugar. I know. They don't tell you that. They also don't tell you that a review of 21 studies published in the *American Journal of Clinical Nutrition* found no clear link between the consumption of saturated fat (found in meat and dairy products) and a higher risk of developing heart disease or stroke. *They* don't tell us a lot of things.

High levels of refined carbohydrates cause our blood sugar to elevate. When that occurs, the liver works to convert that sugar into something it can store. The liver can't store a very large quantity of carbohydrates, so if we eat a lot of carbs, insulin is produced by the pancreas and attaches itself to the sugar and moves it to the liver. The liver converts that sugar into triglycerides, a component of fat. As you know, we have an unlimited capacity to store fat.

The liver does more with triglycerides. It turns them into something called VLDL's, very low density lipoproteins. You've heard of LDL's, the bad cholesterol? VLDL's are worse. They produce the most dangerous lipoproteins which then result in inflammation and plaques in your arteries. They deplete the body of HDL's, the good cholesterol. By the way, HDL 2B is the most beneficial cholesterol.

A complete blood test panel of factors is available from your doctor. It comprises much more than the old total cholesterol and HDL/LDL ratio.

What's neat is that you can lower your triglycerides and thus your risk of heart disease and stroke. How? Stop looking for low-fat. Stop looking for that panacea. Start reducing your refined carbs. Go for the whole foods. Your liver will be happy, and so will your heart.

Using a Statin Drug? Consider CoQ10

IN a previous chapter, I discussed the use of whole foods as the fundamentals in our diets. If you don't get all the variety that you can get from eating whole foods, there are whole food supplements available. I recommend one to all my patients as insurance that they are getting what they need. The vitamin bottle definitely plays second fiddle to whole foods.

However, you should know about a single and very important nutritional component, CoQ10 or Coenzyme Q10. CoQ10 is a naturally occurring compound in the body. It works in each cell to produce energy for that cell to work at an optimum level. We manufacture our own CoQ10, but as we age, we produce less and less of it. CoQ10 provides the source of energy to all of our muscles, including our heart. It, all by itself, has been shown to reduce hypertension. In fact, if you have low blood pressure, CoQ10 may be something that you don't want to take.

CoQ10 was touted as a periodontal treatment adjunct years ago. While I never found it to be particularly effective for most periodontal patients, I did have and continue to have some amazing stories on the use of CoQ10 in my surgical patients. About 20 years ago, I had a patient who wasn't healing well after a relatively minor periodontal surgical procedure. I told her to take CoQ10. In two days, she was nearly completely healed. The same thing happened with another patient three weeks later. CoQ10 has now become a routine part of my pre-operative instructions. And if there are times when patients might not follow this recommendation and they heal a little more slowly than they should, I reinforce the recommendation and most do better. Now this isn't science. This isn't a controlled study. It is an observation.

Many of us have been prescribed statin, or cholesterol-lowering, drugs. One problem with those statin drugs is that they drive our own CoQ10 out of our bodies by as much as 50%. Ever experienced leg cramping while on a statin drug? That may be due to that CoQ10 reduction. Many doctors recommend CoQ10 for their statin patients to help replenish the lost nutrient. In fact, one of the prominent pharmaceutical companies has a patent that combines their statin drug with CoQ10. Unfortunately, it hasn't been put on the market.

There is lots of information on CoQ10 on the internet. One good source is written by a former physician astronaut, Dr. Duane Graveline. You can log on to www.spacedoc.com to see his material.

Don't Wait When Signs of a Stroke Appear

I THINK it was Mark Twain who said, "Denial ain't just a river in Egypt."

Denial of stroke symptoms could mean the difference between function and paralysis, between speaking normally and struggling to get a word out, and possibly between life and death.

There are two basic kinds of strokes. One comes from a blood clot that clogs an artery going to the brain. That is treatable. The other comes from a burst blood vessel in the brain. You can't tell the difference without a CT scan, and the quicker the CT scan is taken, the better.

If you have a clot, there is a lot that can be done to dissolve the clot before it damages the brain permanently. But the clot needs to be dissolved quickly. Otherwise the blood supply to that part of the brain stops, and if that part isn't getting blood, those brain cells will die.

So here's the message: If you suspect a stroke, don't wait. Don't say that it will get better. Don't say that you only need a little time. Don't say it's just a minor thing.

So what are the symptoms of stroke?

- If you suddenly have difficulty walking, you stumble, or your gait changes, that could be a stroke.
- If you have difficulty talking, slurring your speech, or can't get words out, you could be having a stroke.
- If you have paralysis or weakness on one side of the body, including numbness, that's a sign of a stroke. The same holds true if one side of your mouth droops.
- If you have trouble seeing in one or both eyes, that's a sign of a stroke.

- And if you have a sudden, severe headache, that could be a sign of a stroke.

I emphasize that these are immediate changes, changes so significant that you didn't have them the day before, and just because they might temporarily go away is no reason conclude that you're not having a stroke. Those symptoms can come and go.

A stroke center will immediately do those tests necessary to determine if you're having a stroke. All of our major hospitals have stroke centers. The window for successful treatment after a stroke can close as soon as three hours following the stroke, so there isn't much time. There certainly isn't time for denial because if you wait, you simply don't have nearly as good a chance to recover.

Can other problems mimic strokes? Yes, they can, but the only way to know it is to have the problem diagnosed quickly. If you have sudden symptoms, call 911 and get to one of those hospitals quickly. Quick action may preserve your health and even save your life.

Indigestion Is More than a Nuisance

THERE'S this idea that as we age we should be able to eat just as we did when we were teenagers. I went to South End Pizza with my friend Sandy when I was eighteen. I remember it so well because we ordered the largest pizza they had and ate the whole thing. I also remember how I felt the rest of the night. That was the day that I understood that I can't eat everything.

So how about you? Do you try to eat everything? Well, listen: the older we are, the less leeway there is for our digestive tract to handle the foods that we eat. The result of that is "indigestion" and a specialized form of indigestion is called gastroesophageal reflux disease (GERD). Food hits your stomach. Rather than making the traditional path through the digestive system, it comes back up carrying stomach acids along with it. The constant bathing of your esophagus with acid creates damage to the esophagus, called Barrett's esophagus, and can dissolve the enamel of your teeth. If you're dependent on drugs to allow you to eat the way you want, that may produce a bigger problem down the road.

The offenders that I'll talk about today are the proton pump inhibitors (PPI), which are widely prescribed, probably too much so according to some pretty scholarly articles in the *Annals of Internal Medicine*, a widely read medical journal. What's a proton pump inhibitor? Without going into brand names, if the generic name ends in -prazole, it is a PPI. It works by binding stomach acid at the source of its production. Sounds good, doesn't it? But we need stomach acid to digest our food. When that acid level is reduced too much, other problems occur. The big problem that may occur, particularly among the elderly and hospitalized patients, is an intestinal bacterial infection called Clostridium difficile, better known as C diff. The C diff infection is difficult to treat and can be fatal.

Opinions vary on the relationship between PPI's and C diff. A prevalent thought is that we have C diff in our intestines anyway, but it is kept in check by the acids in our stomach. Once we change that acid-base balance, C diff can then proliferate. C diff can be transmitted from person to person. It can also result from the overuse of antibiotics.

But let's go back and look at how we are eating and what we can do to reduce the use of these PPI's. First is to get to the cause of the problem. If you're eating acidic fruits, such as citrus fruits, just substituting a less acidic fruit such as an apple may solve the problem. If you're eating big, heavy meals, you can reduce the problem by eating several small meals a day. There are digestive aids that can be purchased in the health food store that increase your ability to digest your foods, reducing your tendency to develop too much stomach acid. If you're eating a lot of junk, just stop it. And remember, if it's in a can or a box, it's generally highly processed food that your stomach may not know how to handle.

While the diagnosis of GERD or other digestive problems is important, your ability to change your lifestyle to stop the GERD is the real key. Visit a nutritionist. Look online and read some books on GERD. You'll find out some simple things that you can do to stop the reflux. The more you do, the less reliant you will be on medications, and that's how you can improve your overall health.

Gluten Sensitivity

IT'S interesting how many people ask me about my health. People want to see my new veneers and check to see if my warts are still gone (they are). My guess is that they assume that I have the other problems that I talk about in this column. Well, I don't have many health problems, have never had a dental implant done, and haven't taken the medications that I speak about in this column—except for one, and now I'm almost off that entirely.

For years, I had a chronic cough. It worsened and developed into acute bronchitis a few times. Finally, I started using one of those inhalers that you're supposed to use twice a day. That was the only answer that I had, and while I tried alternative means and was able to reduce the frequency of using the inhaler, I still needed it.

Here was a hint that I should have taken more seriously: whenever I had cookies or cake, I would cough a little. My daughter used to chastise me when she worked in my office whenever I would sneak some of those goodies. But I still ate them, and with an office staff of about fourteen people now, it was always someone's birthday or anniversary, and our patients are so generous that they bring in treats as well.

So then I came upon a book, *Wheat Belly*. Written by a cardiologist who suffers from severe gluten sensitivity, *Wheat Belly* covers the history of genetic engineering of wheat, the effects on his patients, and the remarkable responses they had when they stopped consuming all wheat products. Lots of us are sensitive to gluten, and it's not just digestive sensitivity. Have you noticed that gluten sensitivity is a relatively new finding? There's a reason for that. Wheat, which is the source of much of our gluten, has changed. With the magic of genetic engineering, we now have wheat crops that are heartier, have shorter growing seasons, and are not as susceptible to weather and bugs. With that same magic of genetic engineering, 5 percent of the gluten in that wheat has never been seen before. So, would it then make sense that our bodies don't know what to do with this new gluten?

And so it is. Whether it's whole grain or refined flour, it is made up of the same new, *improved* wheat, creating multiple health problems, most notably obesity and diabetes as well as respiratory problems. So I stopped wheat products. My cough got better without medications. My chiropractor gave me some supplements to accelerate the process, and now I might use the inhaler once a month when I slip up.

What a discovery! And on the other side, with all of the governmental regulations we have, don't you think that there should be regulations forcing the chemical companies who create these new, *improved* agricultural products to test them on real human beings before they are released to the public?

Improve your Health– Tap into your Genetics

Rebecca Hunton, M.D.

DO you have "good genes"? Exactly what does that mean? Attractive features? Athletic ability? Are some people born with an unfair advantage? This is a powerful question, especially when we consider the alternative. Can you be doomed by your genetics? How many of us have a family history of autism, bipolar disorder, cardiovascular disease, rheumatoid arthritis, lupus, depression, chronic lyme, cancer, ADHD, miscarriages or strokes? If any of these aliments run in your family, are you destined to suffer the same fate as your elders or can you overcome your genetics? With recent advances in human genetics, we have identified one gene that impacts all of the conditions listed above and if we can identify and "support" its functions, we can significantly lower the risk of all of these conditions.

The gene is MTHFR. No, it's not an expletive. MTHFR stands for MethylTetraHydroFolateReductase, and it controls our ability to methylate. When our body has a reduced capacity to methylate, we are more susceptible to chronic disease.

What is methylate? It is a biochemical reaction that happens in almost every cell of our body. Every chemical we are exposed to, everything we ingest, every byproduct of our metabolism is processed down different biochemical pathways (think of them as highways where all these chemicals travel in our body.) All hormones, pesticides, fertilizers, BPA, many pharmaceutical drugs, mercury and other metals, ALL need the methylation pathway (or highways) to work appropriately for our bodies to handle these chemicals. This is why the MTHFR turns out to be one of our most important pathways. If one or more of these methylation pathways are closed due to our genetics, we have a diminished capacity to move these toxins through our body, and if they get "stuck", we get sick.

We are born with 2 methylation highways, C677T (think I-95) and A1298T (think US1). We get 2 lanes in each of these highways, one from mom, one from dad. I-95 is the most important highway. If we are born without a lane in one of these highways, or worse, without a highway, we aren't able to process these environmental chemicals appropriately. Using the highway analogy, the more 'cars' we are putting on the roads, the more likely we are to have a 'traffic jam' and suffer the consequences.

So are we doomed if our genes diminishes our ability to 'methylate'? No! By providing the body with the appropriate form of folic acid, we can actually 'bypass' the broken highway and help restore the body to health. Additionally, if we know that we have a problem with the MTHFR highway, we are able to be proactive and avoid the chemicals that will overwhelm our ability to process. Fortunately, MTHFR status is easily determined. Most of our major laboratories can run this test with a physician order.

How common is this? Almost HALF of us have at least one lane that is missing in the MTHFR highway system. 50 years ago, that didn't matter because we just didn't have many chemicals traveling those highways. Unfortunately, the majority of the chemicals developed over the last 50 years need methylation in order for the human body to process them safely. If you, or someone you love, is suffering from any of the conditions listed above, seek out a physician to help determine and address their MTHFR status.

Rebecca Hunton, MD has an Integrative medical practice in Viera. She is an expert on the successful application of lifestyle medicine to achieve optimal health and wellness. Dr. Hunton is a preferred provider to members of the NFL Players Association, a member of TEDActive and most notably, her patients have been featured on the Dr. Oz show to demonstrate successful aging with vitality . Her website is drhunton.com

Osteoporosis

OSTEOPOROSIS is a mammoth problem in this country.

Ok, so there's a well-known secret that's advertised on nearly every osteoporosis drug commercial concerning the use of bisphosphonates. You don't pay attention to it until you need the service. What's the warning? "Osteonecrosis of the jaw (ONJ), which can occur spontaneously, is generally associated with tooth extraction and/or local infection with delayed healing, and has been reported in patients taking bisphosphonates...Known risk factors for osteonecrosis of the jaw include invasive dental procedures..."

So here's what I've seen in regard to ONJ. Patients' bones fail to heal properly. They are chronically sore. Little pieces of bone flake away continually for months or even years. And even when we remove the flaking bone, it still doesn't heal well. The quality of the bone has changed. It just doesn't act the way normal bone acts. It doesn't happen all the time, but most of us that do surgery run into these patients in our practices.

In an attempt to reduce the risk of oral surgery in the presence of bisphosphonates, we often ask our patients to take a "drug holiday" of three months before we attempt oral surgical procedures on those patients who have been taking bisphosphonates for over three years and then delay resumption of the drug until all areas are thoroughly healed. But even when we do that, there are some patients who still have a delayed healing response.

Bisphosphonates are the most common drug used for treating osteoporosis. Fosamax, Actonel, and Boniva are the most popular oral bisphosphonates. There are others that are injectable. The package insert will tell you if you are taking a bisphosphonate drug.

How do bisphosphonates work? There are two primary cells involved in bone metabolism. The osteoblast forms new bone, while the osteoclast takes the old bone away. A bisphosphonate stops the osteoclast from working. So that means that old bone remains and new bone is laid down on top of and around the old bone. That's why a bone scan "looks better" after taking a bisphosphonate.

So, not only is osteoporosis a problem, but the treatment is a problem as well. And the problem is not limited only to bisphosphonate drugs. Estrogen-containing drugs have their risks as well.

Calcium has an affinity for estrogen, so the more estrogen, the more calcium. That's good from a bone standpoint and estrogen-containing drugs do not have the same oral surgery risk that bisphosphonate drugs do. But that doesn't mean that they don't have a risk. Increased estrogen is associated with an increased risk of breast cancer.

So what does one do? My overall theme is "Do everything that you can without medication," because if you correct what you might be doing that's bad for your body, the problem may resolve itself.

So, what should you do? Acid levels in the body seem to make a difference in osteoporosis, and alkalizing (non-acidic) foods can make a big difference. Practically all vegetables, as well as eggs, plain yogurt, and beans, are alkalizing. All meat is acid-forming. A little reading on the subject will give you some dietary guidance on acid-forming and alkaline-forming foods. And there's reasonable evidence that adding some sodium or potassium bicarbonate may help restore bone as well.

In addition, natural progesterone cream has very beneficial effects with no reported cancer risk. A study by Dr. John Lee found that adding natural progesterone cream to an already established osteoporosis program increased bone density up to 10 percent in 6 months and 3-5 percent annually until stabilizing at the level of a 35-year-old. The rest of the program included a diet rich in green vegetables, limiting meat to three times a week, and elimination of sodas, alcohol, and smoking. Along with that was 20 minutes of daily exercise, and calcium, vitamin D, vitamin C, and beta-carotene (*Alternatives*, Dr. David Williams)

Yes, the drugs are there. But wouldn't it be great if we correct the cause of the problem in the first place?

Do You Have Warts?

LET'S lighten up for a moment. After all, it's summer. We can talk about dentistry again in a few weeks. Let's talk about a problem that I had and you may have as well: warts, those crusty, pesky, painful things that show up on hands, feet, and other parts of the body. And no, I'm not talking about genital warts.

Okay, so here's the admission. I had warts. I had them for over five years. I froze them with home therapies. I had them frozen at the dermatologist's office four different times. I know that I'm a dentist and I'm not supposed to talk about pain, but let me tell you that freezing warts is more uncomfortable than anything that I do in my office. At least I get my patients numb. I wasn't numb when that wad of cotton filled with liquid nitrogen was placed and held on my warts, one wart at a time. I had three. One of my warts had babies following one of the treatments, so I then had three warts where I had one, a total of five warts. I even went to a dermatologist in Orlando who had a fancy laser that's made specifically to treat warts. You think the freezing was bad? The fancy laser felt like nails were being driven through my finger, again and again, and then he told me that he'd see me in four weeks and we'd do it again. Yeah, right.

Oh, yes, of course I tried the preparations you buy in the drug store. I used an emery board to shave the warts down before applying the medication, which had a combination of salicylic acid and a glue to help it remain in place. It was like placing airplane glue on my fingers, but it didn't smell nearly as good. (Now I know I'll get letters from the anti-glue–sniffing activists.) They still didn't go away. On Sunday night, I developed a routine of shaving the crusty warts down with a safety razor so they wouldn't look so ugly.

My daughter in law, Jenifer, had observed my wart battles. She worked at a hospital in Boston while my son was in dental school. She had a wart, too, and she told me that secret just a few weeks ago. She went to the chairman of the department of dermatology at Harvard Medical School. You know what he told her? "Use duct tape, and make sure you use the brand-name duct tape, 'Duck' duct tape. It has a special glue."

Who was I to argue? My warts were hurting more and more. I was using up razor blades at an ever increasing pace, and sometimes they'd bleed if I shaved them too deeply, and he was the chairman of the department of dermatology at Harvard. Besides that, Jenifer was my daughter-in-law. You have to listen to your daughter-in-law, don't you?

Well, I listened to her. I found Duck duct tape, and to my pleasant surprise, it came in a number of colors. I bought three different colors: traditional silver, hospital white, and the Jimi Hendrix psychedelic color. I figured that one would go with my pink scrubs the best. You've seen my pink scrubs. If I was wearing those, who would ever question 1970s retro tape on my fingers?

Here's what I found: the silver still stuck the best. The tie-dye color still produced questions. But the white? No one said a word.

I was good about wearing the duct tape twenty-four hours a day for three full weeks, changing the tape when it got wet and started peeling off. I had tape at my desk, in my car, and at home. I was prepared to retape whenever and wherever I was. And guess what? My warts are gone. That was well over five years of suffering over in three weeks.

Thanks go to Jenifer. I wonder what change in me she's going to suggest next.

Magnesium May Help Solve Many Chronic Problems

THIS column has at times become an anthology of my health experiences. As a result, you know that I feel that chiropractic works and that I see two different chiropractors for two different things. You also know that I've seen results from a fruit and vegetable supplement, that I avoid wheat products, have mild sleep apnea that I've treated with an oral appliance, and that my warts were cured with duct tape. Sounds like a revival of the magazine True Confessions.

So here's the next one: muscle spasms. Do you wake up with leg cramps? Do you have muscle cramps during the day? I did, and I knew about the solution years ago but ignored it and finally got around to solving the problem. What was the solution? Magnesium.

Magnesium is a mineral. In 1900, our intake of magnesium was about 500 mg a day. Today, the average intake of magnesium is less than half of that. What's happened since 1900? We've removed minerals from our water. Our soil is depleted of magnesium. Our modern processed wheat has most of the magnesium removed. Diets high in refined carbohydrates (sugar) require magnesium for metabolism, so it's depleted even more.

What are the results? Muscle cramps for sure. But then there is high blood pressure and nerve irritability, which can not only result in pain, but also in anxiety. Quite a bit of research points to diminished magnesium as a primary cause of heart attacks, congestive heart failure, and arrhythmias. An example of the effects of depleted magnesium is Finland, which was once the number-one country in cardiac deaths. The country instituted a magnesium supplementation program and the stats quickly dropped to number ten in cardiac deaths.

Magnesium has been linked to symptoms of ADHD. One study of 116 children with ADHD showed that 95 percent of them were magnesium deficient.

So what foods do have magnesium? Bran from rice, wheat, and oats; pumpkin, sesame, and sunflower seeds; Brazil nuts, pine nuts, almonds, cashews, and peanuts; dry-roasted soybeans, kidney beans, and black beans; spinach and other leafy vegetables; and halibut.

A simple blood test for magnesium often won't show deficiencies because only about 1 percent of the mineral shows up in our bloodstream.

The simplest solution, particularly if you have some symptoms, is to take a magnesium supplement. It is inexpensive. I found mine at a large department store. Within a couple of days, my muscle spasms were nearly totally gone. Adult females would generally take about 300 mg a day; males, 400 mg. Personally, I have nuts every day and take 250 mg once a day. Taking the total dosage at one time may produce diarrhea, and it's best if you spread the dosage over the day by taking proportions at meal times.

If you like to take baths, Epsom salt is magnesium sulfate. So you can soak and absorb magnesium at the same time. You'll find Epsom salts at any pharmacy.

Magnesium is safe. It's one of those no-brainers that is inexpensive and could produce dramatic improvements.

[This material was derived from the *Alternatives* newsletter by Dr. David Williams.]

Iodine Is a Necessary Nutrient

I LEARN so much from my patients. And while I spend the vast majority of my time helping to rehabilitate very sick mouths, the fact is that a sick mouth can be an indicator of a sick body. I was having a conversation about that very thing when a patient talked to me about iodized salt. It was then that I knew my next column would be on iodine, because she said that the reason that iodine is in table salt is because it helps with baking.

Iodine may help with baking. I'm a pretty good cook, but I don't bake, so I can't verify that. What I do know is this: Iodine is added to table salt for health reasons. It was a government mandate in the 1920's to add iodine to table salt because of a nationwide iodine deficiency that resulted in enlarged thyroid glands called "goiters." Most goiters are an indicator of hypothyroidism. People ate at home much more often, and salt had no stigma, was a commonly used condiment, and was therefore the best way for our government to help alleviate the goiter problem. And yes, the treatment of iodized table salt worked wonders to eliminate a goiter.

By now, however, we've forgotten the importance of iodine. Our use of iodized table salt decreased by 65% between 1971 and 1994 and it continues to drop. And what do you think is happening as a result? The incidence of goiters and their cause, hypothyroidism, is increasing in the U.S.

You see, the thyroid gland acts as an iodine sponge, and when it doesn't get enough iodine, it gets sluggish and enlarges. When your thyroid gets sluggish, so do you. Some of the problems associated with iodine deficiency include chronic fatigue, weight gain, low metabolism, bone loss, increased cholesterol levels, fat retention, depression, hair loss, intolerance to cold, enlarged thyroid, exhaustion, poor sex drive, and poor circulation.

Other things have changed since the 1920's. We've increased the amount of fluoride and chlorine in our water supplies. Both fluoride and chlorine are chemical antagonists to iodine. So we may need even more iodine now than we did then. And if you have some concerns about increased levels of radiation in our environment due catastrophic nuclear events such as the Japanese nuclear power plant disaster of 2011, one of the products of nuclear fission is radioactive iodine. Your thyroid doesn't recognize the difference between a supplement of inorganic iodine and radioactive iodine. So if you're iodine deficient, which many of us are, the thyroid will absorb what it can get. And radioactive iodine is not a healthy form of iodine.

At the minimum, I'd recommend buying iodized table salt and use it. Personally, I'm taking an iodine supplement. Make sure that it is the inorganic kind, the type that would be found as a supplement, not the kind that's used as an antiseptic, which is poison.

Finally, do some reading on the subject. Dr. Guy Abraham has made iodine his life's work. You can find his material at www.optimox.com.

Vitamin D for the Flu Season

Dr. Lee Sheldon

ANYONE have a doubt that flu season is beginning? It's advertised at pharmacies, on TV, at food stores. There is something that you can do that won't hurt and may very well help you: Take more Vitamin D.

"I thought Vitamin D was for bones," you say. Vitamin D absorption is an adjunct for calcium absorption for sure. But that's only part of it. A pandemic, worldwide Vitamin D deficiency is commonly recognized in the medical literature. In the Mayo Clinic Proceedings earlier this year, there was evidence that deficiency in Vitamin D is related to the following conditions: type 1 diabetes mellitus, cardiovascular disease, certain cancers, cognitive decline, depression, pregnancy complications, autoimmunity, allergy, and even frailty.

What about flu? Dr. John Cannell published a study that shows how important exposure to sunlight is. Our bodies convert sunlight into vitamin D. Flu season begins right after the shortest day of the year when we get the least sun, and it disappears after the longest day of the year. Flu is more common during the rainy season in tropical countries. In Norway, where there is more consumption of vitamin D–containing foods than almost anywhere else, the elderly are less likely to die in winter. A study published in the British journal *The Lancet* showed people over the age of 65 getting a flu shot had no reduced risk of contracting pneumonia, a likely cause of death during the flu season.

So let's get back to Vitamin D. It's commonly deficient and there is good evidence that it can act as an immune booster. More importantly, so many of us are deficient in vitamin D that we are putting ourselves at risk of having some of the problems listed above. Vitamin D is a vitamin that can be checked with a blood test called a 25-hydroxyvitamin D or 25(OH)D test. There are varying levels that are minimally acceptable, depending on whom you read. The U.S. Endocrine Society has stated that a 25(OD)D test of 30 ng/ml is sufficient, but a maintenance level of 40 to 60 ng/ml is ideal.

That means that for most of us, we need to step up our vitamin D intake. We're lucky. We're in Florida. We can take off our shirts and wear shorts. One twenty-minute, full-body exposure of summer sunlight will result in 20,000 IU of vitamin D in our system in 48 hours. If you're dark-skinned, older, obese, or on cholesterol-lowering drugs (vitamin D is converted in our bodies from cholesterol), you'll probably get far less. A sunscreen with an SPF of 8 or greater will reduce your ability to convert sunlight to vitamin D by up to 95 percent.

Of course, there are Vitamin D supplements. Personally, I take 5,000 IUs of Vitamin D a day, and when my blood test is low, I'll take a lot more. The key is to ask your doctor for the blood test. Then do what you need to get your 25(OH)D to at least 30 and preferably 40 to 60. You'll be healthier as a result.

Pain Relief from Low-Dose Naltrexone

FROM time to time, I depart from dentistry to discuss your overall health. The topic that I'm about to talk about is controversial, and I caution you as I always do when I write on medicine that you should consult with your doctor before you consider any changes in your treatment as a result of the data in this column. However, the changes that I have seen have been so dramatic and data is so easily found on the internet that I felt that it was time to share them with you today.

Naltrexone is a drug. It is in a class of drugs known as opioid antagonists and is used to help people with alcohol and drug dependencies keep from resuming those habits. The ordinary dose is 50 to 100 mg per day. This, however, is not an article about those addictions and how to treat them. It is an article about how, for the past 25 years, a 2 to 4.5 mg dose of the same medication has shown other positive powerful effects. It is known as LDN, low-dose naltrexone.

I first found out about LDN during one of my visits to a well-known complementary medicine institute in another state. As I got to know my physician, I asked him about alternative treatments for multiple sclerosis because someone very close to me had been diagnosed with that problem and was in a lot of pain. Traditional treatments hadn't worked for her, despite a great deal of expense and seeing the best people that she could. My physician said, "Have you ever heard of LDN?" That question was one of those "aha" moments. When I told this person with MS about it, she jumped on it, looked at some articles on the Internet, and found a doctor who would prescribe it for her. Her pain relief was remarkable, and while she still had some of the burning pain, she could function again.

Because LDN is a low dose of a generic drug, there is no pharmaceutical money to research this medication, but there are some studies of note that have been published in the medical literature. One case report of three female patients at the University of Utah showed a significant improvement in pruritus (itching) in scleroderma. Another study of forty Crohn's-disease patients at Penn State University showed not only improvement in pain but also evidence of healing of the digestive tract. Pilot studies are showing indications that LDN not only improves pain and disability associated with MS but also may stop the progression of the problem.

In addition, a pilot study on fibromyalgia was done at Stanford University in 2009. Six out of ten patients felt significant pain relief over that found when taking a placebo. A more comprehensive study has been proposed but has not been released as of yet.

The data that in this column is an indicator only. One should weigh the risks and the rewards of any treatment before deciding to undergo that treatment. However, it is safe to say that naltrexone has been around for a long time and has a good track record of safety in full doses. The nuance in these pilot studies and case reports is less than 2 to 4.5 mg of LDN per day may produce significant clinical improvement in pain and in healing of some chronic degenerative problems.

If you would like some references on LDN, please e-mail me at Info@SolidBite.com.

Sjögren's Syndrome May Affect Your Dental Health

THERE is a debilitating disease that affects at least one million people in the United States, mostly women. It is one of those diseases that we just don't hear a lot about, and while not life threatening, it certainly affects your comfort, happiness, and your dental health. It's called Sjögren's syndrome.

Sjögren's syndrome is an autoimmune disease. I know you've heard that term before, and let's define it. We have an immune system composed mainly of white blood cells, called *lymphocytes*, that protect us from disease. Lymphocytes step up their activity when we are attacked by infections, viruses, and injuries. When the lymphocytes have done their job in a normal condition, the body has a braking mechanism to stop the lymphocytes. In an autoimmune disease, the braking system is gone and the lymphocytes go out of control. They attack the body. In the case of Sjögren's syndrome, the lymphocytes attack the salivary glands and the glands that produce tears. In addition, these lymphocytes produce autoantibodies that also damage the salivary and tear systems and may damage other organs of the body including the joints, lungs, kidneys, nerves, thyroid, liver, and brain.

Sjögren's syndrome often accompanies other rheumatic diseases such as rheumatoid arthritis, systemic lupus, scleroderma, and polymyositis.

There may be improved awareness of Sjögren's syndrome as a result of tennis star Venus Williams's announcement that she had the disease when she departed the U.S. Open in September 2011.

Primary Sjögren's syndrome involves the eyes and the mouth. Secondary Sjögren's syndrome means that it is part of a multiple rheumatic disease problem. The diagnosis of primary Sjögren's syndrome includes a small biopsy of the lip, where the lymphocytic invasion can be seen under the microscope.

From a dental perspective, we've talked about the problems of dry mouth in previous columns. Dry mouth creates acids in the mouth, making you much more prone to decay of your teeth. This decay needs to be prevented, and the best way is to keep your mouth moist and your teeth exquisitely clean. Also drop all sugars. There are a number of artificial salivas that you can purchase at the pharmacy. I also recommend to my patients that they rinse out with baking soda and water every few hours. Just mix a tablespoonful of baking soda in 8 ounces of water and keep it with you all day. Rinse for 30 seconds every 3 to 4 hours. The baking soda will neutralize the acid. Rinses and mints with the natural sugar xylitol may also help as xylitol has been shown to reverse tooth decay. You'll need more frequent dental examinations so that if you do develop decay, it can be discovered and treated as soon as possible.

For the eyes, your doctor may recommend artificial tears and for more severe cases, ointments. Anti-inflammatory medications are sometimes prescribed. For secondary Sjögren's syndrome involving the skin, you should add skin lubricants. You may want to add a humidifier to your air conditioning system. Walking and swimming may help to keep muscles and joints flexible as well as prevent further damage.

For more information, contact the Arthritis Foundation at 800-672-0882.

Taking Fear out of the Equation

I JUST returned from a two-day conference. We all do those from time to time, not only to see new concepts but also to become inspired. I love these trips.

I ran into a colleague from another state. Of course, we talked a bit about old times, but then the discussion took a much more pointed stance as he talked with me about how his practice was doing. He was talking to me about how his practice had declined since its peak in 2008. By the way, this is a common theme among members of my profession. In fact, the concern is so prevalent that my office manager, Danyel Joyner, and I are in the final stages of writing a book for my profession on how to manage a periodontal practice in the current times.

In researching the book, I've talked with colleagues in several parts of the country about their concerns as well. Their comments were much the same as my friend's. Do you know what all of those comments had in common? Fear. It usually goes like this: "But if I do so and so, somebody may not like that." That's fear, but if all of your actions are totally ethical, what is the real problem? Operating from fear is a dangerous operation at best.

Patients walking into my office, as you would understand, often come to me in fear.

My office staff is great, every one of them. They are technically excellent; they know their jobs. But do you know what they do best? They take our patients out of fear. A good staff member in any dental office knows how important that is.

How do they do that? They get into communication with their patients, and as they communicate with each other, the fear lifts away. Once the fear lifts away, then those patients are ready for solutions.

So, in speaking with my friend, we discussed first his concerns and got them all on the table. Next was to talk about some solutions that he might apply. The conversation took a different turn, as he was not necessarily ready to implement some of the solutions that I recommended. Why? Because he was afraid of what someone else might think. Ah, fear again. I backed off a bit and found something that he could accept without fear. We spoke a lot over the next couple of days. He learned something. He found some ways to improve his practice. I learned something, too. I learned that we sometimes have to take small steps in order to implement change.

So what about you? Is there something that you need to change, something that you need to improve? Have you been afraid to confront that because of fear? How about writing down the steps that you would need to take to accomplish that change? Can you now do just the first step? If not, can you divide the first step into smaller steps? Now can you do the first step? Congratulations!

Now do the first step. Please e-mail me at Info@SolidBite.com and let me know what happened.

Antidepressants

THIS topic is one that is affecting all of us. It is something that is not talked about enough, but it's something that requires our attention. And if you read this further, you may scratch your head, shake your head, or hopefully, nod in full agreement. This message is dedicated to the overprescribing of psychotropic drugs. Yes, those drugs; the drugs that have been cleverly marketed as a cure for bad moods, changes of seasons, depression, anxiety, and countless other maladies that beset us.

I see it as a dentist, because I need to know my patients' medical histories. And the longer I have been in practice, the more I see these drugs being prescribed.

From a dental perspective, these drugs, as well as many others, cause dry mouth, and dry mouth results in tooth decay. Such tooth decay is difficult to control and often recurs.

But the facts are more insidious than merely tooth decay. The drugs have multiple effects. Weight gain, diabetes, sexual dysfunction, and a host of serious, life-threatening health problems are common effects of these drugs. Moreover, the drugs are often extremely difficult to stop taking, and complete withdrawal from them requires extensive time and doctor supervision. Sometimes, patients and doctors become confused, thinking that the symptoms that occur during withdrawal are a return of the emotional problem when in fact those symptoms are withdrawal symptoms.

Patients are given inappropriate and wrong information, hearing such statements as, "You have a chemical imbalance," when such a statement is blatantly false. Why? There is no credible study showing what a proper "chemical balance" is. There is no test for making such a diagnosis.

In the past few years, several pharmaceutical companies have been fined hundreds of millions and even billions of dollars by the U.S. Justice

Department for the deceptive marketing of these drugs. Several states have successfully filed suits against these companies as well for failing to reveal previously known, major health problems caused by these drugs. And just this past year, two major companies have dropped researching this class of drugs entirely.

Please look very carefully before deciding to take one of these drugs. Read carefully all the effects of such a drug before you decide to take it. Look at all the things that could be causing the emotional problem. Diet? Exercise? An undiagnosed medical problem? Hormonal imbalance? Nutritional deficiency? Do you need someone to talk to? There are lots of non-drug resources to turn to for help.

If you are taking these drugs and want to stop, please don't do that yourself. Get a physician's help. And help yourself by reading a book on the subject. *The Antidepressant Solution,* by Dr. Joseph Glenmullen, is an easy-to-read book that has helped many. If you want to find out more about this subject, log on to the Citizens Commission on Human Rights, cchr.org.

Seniors' and Families' Guidelines on Involuntary Commitment

THERE are certain facts that are unknown to us until a crisis arrives, and while I try to write with a certain amount of levity, this subject has no lightheartedness about it. The fact is that seniors can be and are "Baker-Acted." What is the Baker Act? It is the involuntary commitment of a person to a psychiatric facility. How does that happen? An individual demonstrates an inability "to exercise voluntary control over his or her own symptoms" (mental health symptoms). This can include depression, anxiety, dementia, irritability, aggression, and so on, and in the judgment of the evaluator the subject is deemed an imminent danger to him or herself or to others. Such must be documented with the "nature and extent of the danger posed." The evaluator can be a law enforcement officer, a psychiatrist, a psychiatric nurse, or a psychologist. A person who has been deemed incompetent to consent to treatment will lose that right to consent and will be involuntarily committed.

The second part of involuntary commitment can be involuntary treatment. Involuntary treatment in a psychiatric institution can include psychiatric drugs, electroconvulsive therapy (also known as electroshock treatment), and psychosurgery. Interestingly, involuntary treatment for people in a psychiatric facility is now illegal in Germany, the birthplace of psychiatry, but it is still allowed in the United States.

There are specific things that a person who is involuntarily committed can and cannot do.

1. The person does have the right to file a petition for a writ of habeas corpus to formally request why he or she is being detained.

2. The person does not have the right to refuse the involuntary commitment but does have the right of informed consent regarding the risks and the alternatives to the proposed treatment. If a person strongly objects to a particular form of treatment, the person's guardian / guardian advocate or surrogate/proxy should talk with the patient to determine the reasons for the objections. If appropriate, the guardian / guardian advocate or surrogate/proxy may, based on this information, withdraw his or her consent for the proposed treatment and negotiate a revised treatment plan with the physician.

There may be many reasons why a person may decide not to consent to a particular medication or to any medication ordered by a particular physician or to treatment ordered at a particular facility. The decision as to whether a person is competent to consent is a clinical judgment of his or her capacity to decide, not one based on whether the person does or doesn't provide such consent.

According to the Baker Act, the psychiatric treatment needs to be given in "the least restrictive manner."

What is most important here is that you, I, all of us should be well-prepared for this possibility. If we have appointed a guardian / guardian advocate in advance, such a person can act on our behalf in this unfortunate situation. If there is no guardian, the administrator of the psychiatric facility, upon the recommendation of the psychiatrist, can authorize what is considered "emergency medical treatment."

The guardian should be well aware of your wishes in advance. Suffice it to say that the irreversible effects of psychiatric drugs, shock treatments, and psychosurgeries are well documented. There is no medical test that psychiatry performs to evidence a "chemical imbalance." Therefore any claim that a psychiatric drug will balance chemicals in the brain is pure folly. However suicide, physical illness, aggression, and other maladies are FDA-listed warnings on the psychiatric drugs and have been well documented.

For further information on this subject, log on to cchrflorida.org or call 800-782-2878.

Acknowledgments

MANY years ago, while I was in college and had no idea what my career path would be, I took a trip to the NYU College of Dentistry with my good friend, Sandy Halperin. Sandy was applying to that school, and I just tagged along with him. Sandy's brother, Mark, was a student at the school as well. Sandy knew he wanted to be a dentist. I had an idea that maybe a career in dentistry would be good for me. That trip to NYU convinced me that this was the career path I should take. So I went home, talked to my girlfriend at the time and soon to be my wife, Eleanor, and let her know that I had decided on dentistry as a career.

Two years later, I was a student at Tufts University School of Dental Medicine. I found dental school to be challenging, but got the hang of it. I knew that I needed and wanted more training, so off I went to Fort Sill, Oklahoma as a general practice resident. It was there that I studied directly under specialists in every field of dentistry. Colonel Brent Ward made a major impact on me as he taught me denture principles that I have carried with me through my private practice. But Dr. Bill Parker showed me what a periodontist was and what a periodontist could do. He emphasized not only treatment, but thinking a case through from start to finish. He loved being the dental consultant that the specialty of periodontics provides.

However, I still had two more years to serve in the army, which I did at the Army War College at Carlisle Barracks, Pennsylvania, where I practiced with three colleagues on the "cream of the crop" in the army. My patients were top-level officers who were taking a year to advance themselves and their careers at the senior service school in the army. They were motivated to advance their careers, and they finally had the time to do the dental work that they had been putting off while on active service, and I was given the opportunity to be their dentist. This gave me the chance to do major reconstructive dentistry only a year out of dental school.

I then attended the University of Connecticut, studying under some of the most prominent biological researchers in our field. Our chairman, Dr. Paul Robertson, went on to become the dean of a major dental college at the University of Washington. Our periodontal microbiologist, Dr. Ken Kornman, went on to become a major force in our field, and is now the editor of The *Journal of Periodontology*, the most significant journal in our field. Two other faculty, Dr. Clarence Trummel, a periodontist and pharmacologist, and Dr. Mark Patters, a periodontist and immunologist, went on to become chairmen of periodontal departments as well. Our visiting faculty gave us clinical training to balance out our biological training, but it was the biological training that made the difference, because we had to think through our cases based upon biological research, not just on clinical techniques.

So with that background, Eleanor and I moved to Melbourne, Florida in 1980 and started a practice limited to periodontics. We were busy from the start. What a great fortune for us. During that time, we made friends within and outside of dentistry. We became active in religious and secular activities. We moved to Melbourne with our first child, Daniel, who is now a professional television sportscaster. And we had our second and third children, Stephanie and Matthew. Stephanie went on to become a police officer and then became my marketing director. I rely on Stephanie for online and media communications as well as transcription. Matthew has completed dental school at my *alma mater*, Tufts University, and is completing an Advanced Education in General Dentistry program at Baylor University. He will be a great dentist and will practice in Melbourne soon. He created a valuable chapter in this book on crown restorations.

Other opportunities arose as a friend, Jim Cain, asked me to be the host of a local television program, *Check Up*. Little did I know at the time that the program would last over eight years and give me the opportunity to meet and interview health professionals from all over our local community and beyond. I learned from my guests. I learned from my bright and delightful co-host, Dr. Petra Schneider, a plastic and reconstructive surgeon. I needed to read up on things just to keep up with her as well as our guests. Dr. Sal Martingano continued the process, asking me to co-host a radio program on psychiatric abuse, where I was able to interview experts from all over the country courtesy of our dynamite producer, Laurie Anspach of the Citizen Commission on Human Rights of Florida.

I learned traditional medicine. I learned the tenets of alternative therapies and befriended Dr. Michael Farley, who taught me principles of naturopathic medicine, as well as how traditional and alternative medicine can be combined to provide the best treatment for the patient. I learned the advantages found in many fields, including chiropractic, acupuncture, herbal therapies, homeopathic medicine, and other areas. I began reading newsletters, such as Dr. Julian Whitaker's "Health and Wellness Letter" and Dr. David Williams' "Alternatives" newsletter as well as many others. And the more I read, the more I was able to help my patients.

Whenever I needed business guidance, the folks at Silkin Management in Portland, Oregon were always there to help me as well as to train my staff and myself in communication, ethics, and organization as well as handling "life in the fast lane."

The current mode of my practice is not what I ever would have expected. I grew to enjoy the transformations that our patients, who were in every sense dental cripples, achieved. People who had once been embarrassed by their dental condition could smile, could date again. Some were able to get better jobs. And suddenly, they were able to eat and chew again. And through the skill and kindness of my staff, there are many who had previously given up on dental care that are now strong ambassadors of what dentistry can do. With the marketing background that I probably originally got from my father, I began to let people know of my interest in helping the worst of the worst dental cases, and after sitting on the name for several years, I called the service "Solid Bite."

There have been many who have helped me achieve this level of service. My wife, Eleanor, has been with me every step of the way, raising our kids, running our dental continuing education organization, The Brevard Study Club, maintaining the finances of the office, and keeping me in order, and I thank her for that. When we were in college, she used to type my papers and made suggestions to me as she typed. We relived our college days through this book as it was Eleanor who did the final review of the manuscript.

My office manager, Danyel Joyner, has that unique perspective of seeing things for what they are, finding the best possible scenario for those things, and communicating them to patients and to staff. And she sweetly keeps me going in the right direction. As I write this, she is pushing me to get this book done on deadline.

Rebecca Caudill, my hygienist of 27 years, has been a Godsend to me and, more importantly, our patients. Rebecca is so skilled as a hygienist that she's solved many patients' periodontal problems in a way that eliminated the need for surgery.

So many people tell me how wonderful my staff is. This staff includes Laura, Nicole, Courtenay, Stephanie, Kasey, Jennifer, and Joy. Here is a group of professionals who love coming to work, working with patients, and seeing the results of their work. Any dentist, any boss, would be thrilled to work with just one of these individuals. What a lucky guy I am.

I was given an additional opportunity from Joe Steckler, former executive director of the Brevard Alzheimer's Foundation and now President of Helping Seniors of Brevard County, to write for the "Focus on Seniors" column for *Florida Today*. He has also kindly made me a featured guest on his radio and television programs. This book is a compilation of the writings that I have done over the past several years as I tried to educate our patients in the logic of my profession as well as the current research and clinical findings, both in dental and overall health care. Thanks, Joe, for providing me with a new dimension to my career.

Dr. Charles Martin, one of my consultants, thought that our patients would benefit from seeing my ideas professionally printed. He suggested that I consult with an editor. Jude Pedersen has been outstanding in making this document more coherent and readable.

I am so pleased that three doctors have chosen to collaborate with me in this book. Dr. Colin Richman, who wrote the foreword to the first book, has done cutting edge research on tooth-bone relationship which I predict will revolutionize orthodontic care. He and I have been friends and colleagues for our entire careers. His patients are so fortunate to have such a thinking being as their periodontist. Dr. Rebecca Hunton is an MD that looks far beyond traditional medicine for answers. It takes a brilliant and caring individual to command respect from both the traditional and alternative health communities. She does just that.

Dr. Matthew Sheldon has added a great deal of breadth not only to this book but to our practice. What a joy it is to work side by side with my son. I've had the distinct advantage of having a referral practice for the majority of my career. Years ago, I counted over 100 dentists and physicians who had referred patients to me for dental implant and periodontal care. I thank them not only for their referrals but for the skill that they exercise in creating great dental solutions for our patients.

There are many who are unrecognized and who have provided material for this book. And they are the patients in my practice. They are why I do what I do, and they are whom I have learned from the most. Thanks to all of you for making my career the most satisfying one could possibly enjoy.

Lee N. Sheldon, DMD

Acknowledgments for *The Ultimate Mouth Manual, Second Edition*

WHAT amazing changes that have occurred in just two years since the first edition of *The Ultimate Mouth Manual* was published! The entire goal of the first edition was to provide a book about dentistry that our patients could understand. It was a dream of mine, one that began when I was a dental student. I was watching The Tonight Show with Johnny Carson when I saw a dentist, Dr. Sydney Garfield, promoting his book, *Teeth, Teeth, Teeth*. I bought that book. Dr. Garfield's message was that we need to make dentistry understandable for the public. Forty years later, there is so much more that dentistry can do, but the plight is the same. Over the years, I have developed an interest in what we can do to improve our overall health. I've added some chapters to round out fundamentals in complementary medicine that I have found valuable to me. I am happy that so many have told me that they read the first book from cover to cover and that they know a lot more as a result.

In the first book, I asked my son, Dr. Matthew Sheldon, to write a chapter while he was in residency at Baylor College of Dentistry after graduating from Tufts School of Dental Medicine, my alma mater as well. Dr. Charles Wakefield was Dr. Matt's mentor at Baylor and was very proud to have an author as one of his residents. My heartfelt thanks go to Dr. Wakefield for writing the foreword to this edition. Now, I'm proud to say that Matthew is in practice with me. What a joy for a father to be able to work closely with his son. Dr. Matt has written several chapters, rounding out a primarily biological book with his passion for esthetics. His wife, Jenifer, works with us, too, although she will be busy raising their first child, Harper Sonnee, who was born just two days ago as I write this. My wife, Eleanor, still runs the business side of the practice as she has since we started the practice. She is a "doctor's wife" who has no hesitation about picking up or dropping off a patient or going to the store to pick up supplies. Our daughter, Stephanie, and her husband, Matt, produced our first grandchild, Gavin Parker Wintercorn, just three weeks ago. Two weeks later, Stephanie is back at the computer, deftly guiding our public relations programs and transcribing our notes from home. So yes, this is truly a family affair. Our son Daniel is now at Comcast Sports Network in Portland, Oregon, providing his viewers with a depth of sports knowledge that will continue to advance his career.

With Dr. Matt aboard, our practice has changed, bringing multiple dental services to our patients all under one roof. It is my long-time friend and office manager, Danyel Joyner, who is guiding that transition, nearly doubling our staff and coordinating expansion of the new phase of Solid Bite. She is a rock to me, making these growth efforts practically seamless. The managers that are working under Danyel—Courtenay Zambrano, Jennifer Ashley, and Laura Widener—help our patients not only during office hours but on nights and weekends, too. Rebecca Caudill has now been my dental hygienist for twenty-nine years, not only keeping our patients periodontally healthy but also keeping most of them out of periodontal surgery. There is no better hygienist anywhere. Dr. Jennifer Chace, in addition to having her own successful practice with her husband, Greg, is also practicing with us, giving our patients superb talent as well has deep compassion. All together, we now have a staff of seventeen people. I am so fortunate to have such dedication and talent surrounding me.

Joe Steckler asked me to join him several years ago in his quest to help seniors. He leaves no stone unturned to forward this agenda and founded Helping Seniors of Brevard County. He's succeeded in his first goal: to give our seniors education on what they can do to help themselves. Joe has taken me under his wing in that quest and as a result, I am a regular newspaper columnist and a featured guest on Joe's television and radio programs. My columns in *Florida Today* are a part of the substance of this book.

The first edition of *The Ultimate Mouth Manual* was met

with overwhelming enthusiasm from the dental community. More importantly, our patients told us that they now understood dentistry in a way that they never had understood it before. That's so important so that they may make informed decisions. We hope that this expanded volume adds to that depth of understanding as we continue our goal of helping you make the right dental decisions for yourself.

Lee N. Sheldon, DMD

INDEX